Midwives
and
Changing Childbirth

Irene Walton
and
Mary Hamilton

Books for Midwives Press
Books for Midwives Press is a joint collaboration
between The Royal College of Midwives and
Haigh and Hochland Publications Ltd

Published by Books for Midwives Press Ltd, 174a Ashley Road, Hale, Cheshire, WA15 9SF, England.

Reprinted 1995

First edition

ISBN 1-898507-15-5

British Library Cataloguing in Publication Data
A catalogue record for this book is available from the British Library

Printed in Great Britain by Cromwell Press Ltd

Dedication

To the women of the future who will use the maternity services
and to Aimee, Hannah, Rebekah and Emma in particular.

Contents

Acknowledgements

We would like to acknowledge and thank our husbands and families for their long-suffering and patient support.

We also wish to express our appreciation and gratitude to colleagues for their helpful comments and particularly to Meryl Thomas, Director of Midwifery Education and Supervision, English National Board, Carole Whewell, Senior Midwifery Manager, Obstetrics, Gynaecology and Paediatric Services, St Helens and Knowsley Hospitals Trust and Catherine Bryant for their critical readership.

Finally, to Henry Hochland for his belief in us.

This book represents our interpretation of the reports and of 'Changing Childbirth' in particular and the views expressed herewith are ours and ours alone. We do not claim to be definitive or representative of any organization or institution.

Introduction

Throughout the 1970s and 1980s it appeared that technology was rapidly taking over the care of the childbearing woman. Midwives were becoming little more than technicians in the process, and the woman herself was becoming unnoticed in the pursuit of the visibility and importance of the fetus. Midwifery in the 21st century was visualized in a highly sophisticated, controlled environment where women were merely recipients of care. In the search for the perfect human being the specialists would have control of the entire process. Midwives as the practical mechanics would have the responsibility to ensure that communication channels to and from the appropriate specialist would be maintained throughout.

What was not taken into account in the equation was the voice of women both as mothers and midwives. Apprehension about this prophecy of the future led to the articulation of voices of dissent firstly from individuals and then from representative groups. Gradually this dissent became a groundswell of opinion as more and more people added their voices to the throng.

As two midwives living through this era, and its inherent frustrations, the possibility of reports such as 'Winterton' and 'Changing Childbirth' seemed beyond the realms of probability. However, the philosophies of respect for the individual, the market economy, individual choices, personal responsibility and consumer satisfaction intersected at a crucial point in time to bring about a climate for change.

'Changing Childbirth' represents a unique opportunity for all professionals involved in the delivery of maternity care to work together to enable women to have choice, control, continuity and ultimately, satisfaction with their experiences during a time of great social, psychological, spiritual and physical change. Midwives, as the main providers of care are uniquely placed to ensure that not only the letter but the spirit of the report is taken forward to a more humanistic future. This opportunity will not present itself again and so must be seized and acted upon by every midwife and by everyone involved in the purchasing and provision of maternity services.

CHAPTER ONE

Background

The Government announced, in its response to the Select Committeee's report, that it would set up an expert Committee: 'to review policy on NHS maternity care, [particularly during childbirth] and to make recommendations' (Department of Health, 1993a, p. 1, no. 5).

The Department of Health has published the most exciting and revolutionary report affecting the maternity services this century. It is 'Changing Childbirth', the Report of the Expert Maternity Group (Department of Health, 1993a) which focuses on the needs and wants of women as recipients of the maternity service and is 'an agenda for change' (Page, 1993).

It not only suggests the changes which are required to develop woman centred care but contains specific targets for action and time limits for their achievement by both the purchasers and providers of the internal market system of the National Health Service. The report of the Expert Group, 'Changing Childbirth' is the culmination of a lengthy process which brought together the strands of ideas, opinions, suggestions and recommendations from many individual professionals, users of the maternity services and organizations with an interest in the maternity services.

The Government regularly sets up inquiries into health matters and the maternity service is no exception. It was over ten years since the Social Services Committee chaired by Renee Short had examined the maternity service in depth (House of Commons, 1979–80) and 'there were voices saying that all is not well with the maternity services and that women have needs which are not being met'. (House of Commons, 1991–92, p. v)

This being so it was decided to set up a Select Health Committee to inquire into the state of the maternity service. Such a Committee is appointed to examine the expenditure, administration and policy of the Department of Health and consists of 11 members with power to require people to give evidence, appoint people with technical knowledge, communicate with any other Committee and meet for the purpose of producing a report to Parliament. In this case the Committee was set up on Monday 21 January 1991 and comprised the following members: Mr Nicholas Winterton (Chairman), Mr Tom Clarke, Mr James Couchman, Mr Jerry Hayes, Mr David Hinchcliffe, Alice Mahon, Sir David Price, Mr Andrew Rowe, Mr Roger Sims, Rev. Martin Smyth, and Audrey Wise. Mr Jerry Hayes was later replaced by Sir Anthony Durant and the committee began its inquiry in April 1991.

Before considering the work of the Committee which culminated in the 1991–92 House of Commons Health Committee Second Report on the Maternity Services (House of Commons, 1991–92) or the Winterton report as it was commonly known, a brief look at the preceding decade and the matters which were causing concern is in order.

The decade opened with the publication of the 'Short report' as the second report from the Social Services Committee (House of Commons, 1979–80) on Perinatal and Neonatal Mortality was commonly known. It agreed unequivocally with the Peel Committee's report of 1970 (Maternity Advisory Committee, 1970) which recommended that small isolated obstetric units should be phased out and be replaced by consultant/general practitioner units in general hospitals and that there should be a 100 per cent hospital confinement rate. The Short Report recommended that home deliveries should be phased out. However it did recognize that the skills of the midwife should be made better use of and also that for the woman was an ideal to be aspired to. It stated that:

> Midwifery is the cornerstone of British obstetric practice yet it is our impression from the evidence we have taken that never in this century, has morale amongst midwives been at such a low ebb.

and

> We recommend that every effort is made to re-establish midwifery as a profession that offers attractive prospects to young women interested in a nursing career. (House of Commons 1979–80, p. 76)

In Chapter 15 it identified a need for the maternity services to become more humanized because it did not consider it enough to concentrate solely on the physical well-being of the mother and her baby.

> The emotional support provided by the maternity services, although more difficult to define, is also of major importance. (House of Commons, 1979–80, p. 91).

So the scene was set for the professionals within the maternity services to look at ways in which the mother and her family could be treated with more warmth and compassion than before.

Following the Short Report the Government set up the Maternity Services Advisory Committee which produced three reports (Maternity Services Advisory Committee, 1982; 1984; 1985) which were to be very influential in the planning of maternity care in the 1980s. They were Maternity Care in Action Part 1 – Antenatal care, Part 2 – Care During Childbirth and Part 3 – Care of the Mother and Baby. These reports were used as guidelines by Maternity Service Liaison Committees, Heads of Midwifery Service, obstetricians and Health Authorities in order to improve the standards of maternity care. The reports also maintained that the best place to have one's baby was in the maternity unit and so hospital confinement was again reinforced as being the safest and best type of care. This was not agreed by everyone and one of the most eminent dissenters in the field was Marjorie Tew (1990) who highlighted the fact that statistically a causal relationship could not be found between the fall in the perinatal mortality figures and hospital confinement. She says:

> The correlation which obstetricians and others claim between increasing medical care, or specific obstetric interventions, and decreasing mortality are quickly shown to be spurious. They all fall at the first hurdle, so that further analysis is never necessary. (Tew, 1990, p. 196)

Other people emphasized that there was more to consider than solely the perinatal mortality rate, for example, Sheila Kitzinger who pointed out that,

> A good birth is not just a matter of safety, or of achieving the goal of a live and physically healthy mother and baby. We want birth to be as safe as possible but should not take it for granted that delivery in an operating theatre is the best way to achieve this. (Kitzinger, 1991, p. 9)

These views were endorsed by both consumer and professional organizations such as the National Childbirth Trust, the Association for the Improvements in Maternity Services and the Royal College of Midwives. For example:

> The maternity services must respond to the social, emotional and education needs of the mother as well as her physical health. Women must be full partners in their care. (*Towards a Healthy Nation*, RCM, 1987. Summary, Chapter 2, 7, para 2.1)

The Association of Radical Midwives (ARM) was in many ways the organization that highlighted the frustration felt by many midwives and mothers with the segmented pattern of care and the lack of support for midwives as autonomous, accountable practitioners in their own right. In 1986 ARM published its proposals for the future of the maternity services in a document entitled, 'The Vision' (ARM, 1986). 'The Vision' which had been devised by a working party of midwives set out basic principles which were eventually taken on board by both the Winterton and Changing Childbirth reports. These were:

- That the relationship between mother and midwife is fundamental to good midwifery care (20).
- That the mother is the central person in the process of care (21).
- Informed choice in childbirth for women (22).
- Full utilization of midwives' skills (23,24).
- Continuity of care for all childbearing women (24a,25,26).
- Community based care (6,15a,20).
- Accountability of services to those receiving them (4).
- Care should do no harm to mother and baby.

(ARM, 1986, p. 2).

This was also the decade in which the NHS underwent many reforms culminating in the internal market as enshrined in the NHS and Community Care Act 1990 (Department of Health, 1990a). A constant theme running through these reforms was the committment to quality and consumer choice and participation. Directives such as 'Patients First' (Department of Health, 1982), the Patient's Charter (Department of Health, 1991) and the Maternity Services (Department of Health, 1994), the Children Act (Department of Health, 1989), Health of the Nation (Department of Health, 1992a) and A Strategy for Nursing (Department of Health, 1989) made this committment evident.

The Select committee 1992–93 took evidence in the form of 446 memoranda from individuals or organizations which included individual midwives, mothers, individual obstetricians, the Royal College of Midwives, the Royal College of Obstetricians and Gynaecologists, the Department of Social Security, the College of Anaesthetists, the Department of Health, the Neonatal Nurses Association, the Foundation for the Study of Infant Deaths, the United Kingdom Central Council for Nursing, Midwifery and Health Visiting (UKCC), and the Association for the Improvement of the Maternity Services, to mention but a few.

The Winterton report was divided into six chapters which looked at policy developments in the maternity services, what women actually want, the evidence from the professionals, the Regional services, the maternity services of the future, and the way forward.

The first chapter traced the policy developments affecting the maternity services from the beginning of the century to the inauguration of the Health Committee itself. It reminded the reader of the appalling mortality statistics at the beginning of the century when the infant mortality rate was 154 per 1000 live births in 1900 as compared with 8.4 per 1000 in 1990 and the maternal mortality peak rate of 4.6 per 1000 births in 1934 compared with 0.081 per 1000 births in 1990. The reader was taken through the resultant reports in a succinct and precise manner which traced the changes in the pattern of care and service provision from the tripartite service of a domiciliary based midwifery service, general practitioner and hospital based care to the integrated service of today. It discussed how the Guillebaud Committee (House of Commons, 1955–56) was set up to review the current cost of the Obstetric Service under the

National Health Service and how it had reported that the Maternity services were in a state of confusion. The Guillebaud Committee also reported that the ultimate aim should be to provide obstetric beds for all women who needed or would accept institutional confinement. As a result of that report the Maternity Services Committee was set up under the Earl of Cranbrook to review the organization of the maternity services. It recommended amongst other things that there should be a 70 per cent hospital confinement rate, but affirmed the right of the midwife to participate in the maternity care of her patients to the fullest extent. The Cranbrook report was followed by the Peel Report in 1970 (Maternity Advisory Committee, 1970) which went further and recommended 1005 hospital confinement, the rationale being that,

> The greater safety of hospital confinement for mother and child justifies this objective. (House of Commons, 1970)

The Winterton Report continued to trace the development of the Maternity Service to date and looked at the recommendations of the Short Report (House of Commons, 1979–80), the Maternity Services Advisory reports – Maternity Care in Action Part 1.2 and 3 (1982,1984,1985) and the evidence from individuals such as Marjorie Tew (1990). After looking at the evidence it concluded that encouraging all women to give birth in hospital cannot be justified on the grounds of safety and that the pattern of maternity services or care should not be driven on a medical model of care based on unproven assertions.

Chapter 2 of the report looked carefully at the issues surrounding what women want and need, in particular the aspects of continuity, choice and control by women in childbirth. Evidence from many consumer organizations, such as the Maternity Alliance, led the committee to conclude that there is a strong desire amongst women for continuity of care and that midwives are the best group to provide this. On consideration of the choice of treatment and the place of delivery it felt that choice was often more illusory than real. Consumer organizations told the committee that there was little real choice because of institutional factors and the push towards 100 per cent hospital confinement. The committee were of the mind that the present structure of the maternity services actually frustrates rather than facilitates women who wish to choose.

Another strong theme running throughout the chapter was that of control and participation. Women need to have choice and it has to be informed choice with women being given 'sufficient, balanced non-judgemental and appropriate information at each stage of the maternity process' (House of Commons, 1991–92, p. xvii)

This need for information was a constant feature with the emphasis always on the woman's needs and preferences. In this way various topics such as the work of link workers, the place of confinement, breastfeeding, and care after bereavement were examined in order to make recommendations on best practice. Overall the evidence showed that women were in accord in wanting emotional support, continuity of care, a confident and confidence inspiring birth attendant and choice and control over their own bodies.

After taking evidence from the women about what they want the Report looked in Chapter 3 at the evidence from the professionals about what they believe women want. The main evidence came from the three Royal colleges , the Royal College of Midwives (RCM), the Royal College of Obstetricians and Gynaecologists (RCOG) and the Royal College of General Practitioners (RCGP). The Committee felt that the evidence from the three colleges was not as clear and unanimous has it had been from the women. They seemed to be more concerned with which group should have control over the maternity services and the interprofessional rivalries were all too evident.

The Association of Radical Midwives (ARM) identified the medical model of care as being the main impediment to the delivery of team midwifery and a 'midwifery led' service. The RCM stated that women have the right to be full partners in their care and midwives have the right to practice their profession in a system that makes full use of their skills. They pointed out that accepting the 'right' of any one profession may take precedence over the needs of mothers.

The RCOG did state that midwives should be able to give intrapartum care for women in the community but according to the report (p. xxxvi) they had not confronted the practical implications for the organization of the maternity services. Most of the witnesses from the RCOG did not cite continuity of care or mothers' satisfaction when asked to give their criteria for good maternity care. However Professor Beard did say, that it is no longer acceptable to provide that care without the informed agreement of pregnant women and their partners. (House of Commons, 1991–92, p. xxxvii)

This was also echoed in the report by other members of the RCOG.

The RCGP acknowledged the growing demands for women to have control over their own pregnancy and childbirth for continuity of care and further acknowledged that the system of maternity care was falling below the ideal. They thought that the general practitioner was the professional best placed to provide continuity of care. The members of the Committee detected in the evidence of the RCGP a continuing adherence to a medicalised and paternalistic pattern of service delivery.

After listening to the evidence of the professionals the Committee were not convinced that the organization of the maternity services had succeeded in resolving the conflicts between the various philosophies of care. It went on to look at various aspects of care and made several recommendations aimed at improving practice and developing research-based practice.

Although the focus of the report was mainly upon pregnancy and childbirth as normal physiological events it reminded the reader in the fourth chapter that sometimes events do not proceed normally and mothers and babies may sometimes need highly skilled and specialized medical attention. This is usually provided by regional services and so the Committee looked at these services. From the evidence presented it was persuaded that the overall success of the maternity services depended upon having an efficient and effective backup regional service. This being so its recommendations were to those that would enhance the care, e.g. it recommended that ill babies requiring intensive care should not be refused admission nor should twins or higher order siblings be separated and sent to different hospitals. It also concluded that in this period of change the regional specialities should be protected.

When considering the maternity services of the future in Chapter five, the committee concluded that the philosophy 'no birth is normal except in retrospect' is an impediment to the delivery of a maternity service that meets the needs of the women it serves. It felt that the time had now come for a shift in the emphasis and in the development of policy for the maternity services. It acknowledged that it needs energy, determination and leadership at all levels in the National Health Service and the Department of Health to bring about a climate in which the needs of the women are assessed and met. This being so the Committee recommended a radical reappraisal of the system with a presumption in favour of abandoning shared care. The report also recommended that small units should not be closed on the grounds of safety and that they should remain as an option for women. Other recommendations were made such as the development of a paramedic facility in order to improve safety and to give women true choice. Further precise recommendations such as improvement of the environment of the delivery suite were made which again were aimed at improving the experience of women emotionally as well as obstetrically. The Committee were well aware of the financial implications of their report and recommended that sufficient funds were put aside by the Trusts to make full provision for the service. Team midwifery was recommended as a way of providing for women and as a best practice model. Because this was acknowledged to require great commitment from midwives the Committee were anxious that midwives were not deskilled and that the status of the profession was acknowledged. Midwives should also have their own caseloads and the opportunity to establish and run their own midwifery managed units both within and without hospitals.

This chapter was very detailed in its vision of the way forward and looked at many aspects including the financing aspects of maternity care by general medical practitioners, how general practitioners remove women from their lists, and general practitioners as fund-holders. It also considered Purchasing Authorities and the manner of funding maternity care. It considered that consultant posts should be increased after evaluation of factors such as the extra workload due to the reduction in junior doctors hours. In fact it recommended that junior doctors work no more than 72 hours per week. When considering staffing issues it was anxious to ensure that the medical staffing levels targets for the provision of care for newborn infants in regional and subregional perinatal units were achieved as quickly as possible. Overall it aimed at ensuring:

> That the woman having a baby should be seen as the focus of care; and that the professionals providing that care should

identify their needs and develop arrangements to meet them which are based on full and equal co-operation between all those charged with her care. (House of Commons, 1991–92, p. lxxx)

Having considered the shift in emphasis that the Committee wished to see in the underlying philosophy, organization and delivery of the maternity service the Report made it clear in the final chapter that it was not a blueprint for the future because the history of organisation showed that many of the problems were due to a rigid and inflexible approach. The Committee considered that the time had come to turn vague promises of a reappraisal of the maternity service into a programme for action at national level. It concurred with the RCM that this could only happen if there is a determination at the centre to focus attention on the issues raised in the report and to prompt management at local level.

The Committee believed that the three publications of the Maternity Services Advisory committees should be withdrawn and that the NHS Management executive establish a Health Planning forum which should be charged with the specific duty of establishing a national protocol which identifies the targets for the maternity services in terms of health care. This forum would also require health service purchasers to produce specific plans for meeting those targets.

In addition the report looked at the education, research, evaluation and audit issues surrounding good practice in the maternity services. It concluded that there should be a review of the training needs of midwives and general practitioners in the resuscitation of new born babies and an urgent review of the training needs of senior house officers should be undertaken. Midwifery should be afforded the same rights as other professions over the control of its education. Funding for the Medical Research Council should be sufficient to support a full research programme relevant to the maternity services and there should be a midwifery research funding body set up to enable the expansion of research by midwives. The final recommendations were aimed at increasing initiatives that will give information and statistical evidence in order to evaluate maternity care and strengthen the Maternity Services Liaison Committees.

The Winterton Report found much to criticise about the maternity services and blamed medical, midwifery and management professionals as well as politicians and civil servants but it also found great resources of goodwill, skill and commitment to draw upon and it acknowledged in particular the skill of the midwife, the obstetrician and the paediatrician. However it emphasized the need for a dialogue between the resourcers and providers of the service with the users. Above all it affirmed,

> that the needs of mothers and babies are placed at the centre, from which it follows that the maternity services must be fashioned around them and not the other way around (House of Commons, 1991–92, p. xciii).

The Government in its reply to the report (Department of Health, 1992b) affirmed that it will continue to build on the established excellence of the NHS maternity and neonatal services and remain convinced that the safety of the mother and child is of overriding importance. It also pointed out the number of initiatives aimed at improving the maternity services and the care of the newborn that were in place. These included amongst others, the 'Local Voices' initiative, the setting up of a national Confidential Enquiry into Stillbirths and Deaths in Infancy, the Joint Breastfeeding Initiative and the Clinical Standards Advisory Group. Overall the reply was supportive to the report and referred particularly to the task force led by the NHS Executive, which has as its remit the dissemination of good practice in the management of maternity care. The Government's objective for the maternity services is to improve further the information that women have about the options for care and delivery so that they are able to make informed decisions (Department of Health, 1992b, p.5). It did not agree with all of the report's recommendations particularly in the area of finance, for example:

> **recommendation 10** ... that the position of women working in low paid jobs be evaluated to determine whether Family credit should be extended in pregnancy. **2.3.15** The Government believes that to pay Family Credit in such circumstances would be contrary to the primary purposes for which that benefit exists. (Department of Health, 1992b, p.13)

The Government did, however, decide to establish an expert committee to review policy on care during childbirth and to make recommendations.

Also in July 1992 the three Royal Colleges (RCOG, RCM, RCGP) published their report, 'Maternity Care in the NHS A Joint Approach' (RCOG, 1992) which had been in production at the same time as the Winterton report. It presented a framework for maternity care which emphasized 'that the three colleges exist to promote excellence in the interest of those we serve, in pursuit of this objective we know that working together and addressing problems together are the only ways forwards' (RCOG, 1992). It also confirmed the spirit of Winterton and the Government's reply in its statement that,

> Care is best structured as an equilateral triangle with the pregnant woman at its centre. (RCOG, 1992, p.4)

The time was right and the stage set for the creation of the Expert Maternity Group which was to report in detail on the way forward for the Maternity Service, and its report entitled 'Changing Childbirth' (Department of Health, 1993a) was published at the beginning of August 1993.

CHAPTER TWO

The 'Changing Childbirth' Report - An Interpretation

'Pregnancy is a long and a very special journey for a woman ... Maternity services should support the mother, her baby and her family during this journey with a view to their short-term safety but also their long-term wellbeing'. (Department of Health, 1993a p. ii)

The Government in its reply to the report of the Select Committee on Health (House of Commons, 1991–92) announced that it would set up an expert group, the purpose of which was:

'to review policy on NHS maternity care, particularly during childbirth, and to make recommendations'.(House of Commons, 1992)

This it did and the group was set up in October 1992 under the chairmanship of Lady Cumberlege, Parliamentary Under Secretary of State for Health. The Group was composed of ten members including Baroness Cumberlege. They were: Mary Anderson, a senior obstetrician and Gynaecologist; Simon Court, a consultant paediatrician; Peter Farmer, a management consultant; Eileen Hutton, the chairman of the National Childbirth Trust; Liz Lightfoot, a journalist; Lesley Page, a professor of midwifery; Kulbir Randhawa, the coordinator/counsellor of the Asian Family counselling service; Pat Troop, the Chief Executive, Cambridge Health Authority and Cambridgeshire FHSA and Gavin Young, a general practitioner.

The group took nine months to complete its work during which time it visited a variety of consultant maternity units, small maternity units and midwifery schemes. It gathered evidence from a wide range of organizations, professional groups and individuals. A consensus conference was also organized at the Kings Fund Centre in London in March 1993 which was attended by 400 people who were instrumental in the development by the panel of a consensus statement which,

> 'clarified issues and highlighted concerns' (Department of Health, 1993a, p. 2)

In addition the Group commissioned a MORI Health Research study of mothers who had given birth in England since 1989. Women of Asian and Afro-Caribbean origin were also canvassed for their particular perceptions of the maternity services. The Group also commissioned a study by SWT Communications which in addition to identifying the principles of good communication also identified examples of good practice.

The report of the Group was published in August 1993. It identified key aspects of care delivery, namely, that care should be woman-centred, appropriate, accessible and the service should be effective and efficient.

Woman-centred care

The Expert Group was in agreement with the Winterton Report that women and their needs must be at the centre of the care and purchasers and providers must develop maternity services over a five year period to achieve woman-centred care. This being so the Group had to consider what it is that women actually need and want.

It recognizes that each woman has unique needs derived from her medical, ethnic, cultural, social and family background, and a service which is sensitive to those needs is required. To achieve this, facilities for care should be locally accessible and relevant to the population served. Women should be able to gain, within their locality, information about the available services, and also have a choice whether to contact the midwife or general practitioner when first presenting for care. Each woman should have an identified local midwife who will be available for help and advice should this be required. In many instances this midwife will take lead for the planning and provision of care in conjunction with the woman taking into account her expressed wishes. However there will be flexibility in that the lead professional may change as circumstances dictate.If a change in lead professional is required, involvement of the women is necessary so that she feels assured that all professionals involved in care are working together to ensure the best possible outcome for her and her baby.

Antenatal care and visits should be seen by the woman to be relevant to her needs and should take place within the community as far as possible. Throughout her pregnancy the woman should be cared for by people with whom she is familiar and in whom she trusts. The birth plan should be made out when the woman is ready to do so and after she has had enough information to make decisions . Even so, the woman must know that there is the flexibility to change her plans and to know that the professionals will respect her right to choose. The care plan must be individually tailored to her needs.

During her labour the woman should be cared for by people familiar to her and should be made to feel that 'her psychological and physical needs are understood, her privacy is maintained and her autonomy respected' (Department of Health, 1993a, p. 6). If the woman gives birth in hospital the environment should be such that it can instil a feeling that positive empathetic support is available for her and her birth partner.This will be achieved by staff as well as by the surroundings (Para 1.11).

After the baby is born the woman and her partner should be allowed to relax together with the knowledge that help is at hand,if required In the weeks following the birth, the woman and her family should be aware of the support that is available for them and if the woman delivered in hospital she should have as much information as possible regarding available support on return home.

Appropriate care
Safety

The Group acknowledged that in much of the evidence, there was a great emphasis on safety in relation to choice. They do, however, make it very clear in the report that safety is a fundamental principle of the care and state 'safety is not an absolute concept.It is part of a greater picture emphasizing all aspects of health and wellbeing' (para.2.1.6) . It must not be used as an overriding principle and an excuse for unnecessary interventions, e.g. as a reason to impose arrangements that mothers find unhelpful and disturbing.

Meeting the needs of individuals

In order to make the woman and their families 'centre stage' (Department of Health, 1993a, p.11) the service will need to be 'flexible and responsive'. Information must be available to ensure that women know how they can approach a midwife or their general practitioner at the outset of their pregnancy. For women whose first language is not English, access to interpretation facilities is essential to ensure that they too have appropriate information.

Concern was voiced in that the professionals may not communicate with each other and the Report emphasizes that a midwife should keep the general practitioner informed and that midwives, GPs and obstetricians should work in a complementary way. It is also stressed that women can, if they so wish, be referred to an obstetrician. All women should have the opportunity to be seen at least once in pregnancy by an obstetrician. The attitudes of professionals comes under scrutiny with the Group stating, 'We are convinced that the most fundamental change that needs to occur is one of attitude' (p.12). While acknowledging that changing attitudes is not easy, it can be achieved. The Expert Group used the example of women holding their own notes, and the resultant breakdown of previously held views regarding the viability of this system..

While the aim should be for a normal physiological labour, there is recognition that complications may occur. If they do, the woman must be referred promptly. Even when complications do occur the woman should be very involved in the decision-making process and should continue as far as possible to be cared for by the named professional throughout. It is also recognized that there may be times when the relationship between the woman and her caregiver may not be satisfactory and it should be possible, with the agreement of the woman, to allocate another provider of care.

Trusted and familiar faces

The Group were told by many women that one of the most comforting factors, especially at the onset of labour, was seeing a familiar face. This was confirmed by the evidence from the Royal College of Midwives, The Royal College of Obstetricians and Gynaecologists, the Royal College of Anaesthetists, the Association for Improvements in Maternity Services, the Maternity Alliance and other groups.The importance of continuity of carer and adoption of 'the lead professional' in ensuring a 'familiar face' is reiterated, whether this be the doctor or the midwife. The Patients Charter (Department of Health, 1991) requires that there is a named midwife for every woman in order to improve continuity of carer. This midwife, wherever possible, should be based in the community so that she can be with the woman when and where needed. This has been reiterated in the Government's response to the Winterton report (House of commons, 1992) and is endorsed by the Expert Group. However where the pregnancy is more complicated the lead professional may be the obstetrician. Because general practitioners already give continuity of care, it is recommended that they be encouraged to develop their skills and experience to enable them to continue to give care during labour (Para 2.3.16).

Over 40 per cent (Institute of Manpower Studies, 1993) of units have turned to team midwifery in order to provide continuity of care. However, the Group noticed that very few teams had actually managed to achieve continuity (as defined by the IMS team). Other attempts at continuity, e.g. domino schemes or group practices are being developed by some providers, but in many instances these need to be refined to develop greater continuity of carer. Some teams are too large to achieve their aims and in some cases the mother now sees more people in the antenatal period than before, e.g. in the antenatal clinic the presence of a team instead of a permanent staff might mean that the mother could see eight midwives rather than two as previously.

Making group practices and team midwifery work will need commitment, planning and flexibility and, in addition, may mean that the terms and conditions of service, including remuneration for the midwife, will need to be reviewed. This will have to be taken on board by the providers in order to make continuity of care a reality. However, the Expert Group states 'that there is considerable empirical evidence' (para. 2.3.18). to indicate that the continued presence of a qualified carer during labour, together with 'reassurance and a comforting touch',have a beneficial effect on the physical and psychological outcome of childbirth. Maternity units should work closely with purchasers, family health services authorities and consumers in order to achieve this aim.

Access to maternity beds

At the moment access to a maternity bed is via consultants or general practitioners willing to provide the service. The group believes that in woman-centred care the woman should have access to maternity beds through whichever professional she books. This being so, midwives should be able to admit women in labour to maternity unit beds.

Reviewing antenatal care

The group found that antenatal care was the area which was least focused, e.g.women complained of being given differing advice by different midwives. There did seem to be a commitment to reducing the number of antenatal visits that women had to make to hospitals but there was little evidence of a fundamental reappraisal of the service and its purpose. Little attention had been paid to the work of Hall (Hall et al, 1980) which showed that over-attendance at antenatal clinics could affect the standard of antenatal care given, in that time spent undertaking unessential examinations could be better utilized to give more individual and appropriate care to all women. Even in uncomplicated pregnancies the Group found that 12–14 visits was not uncommon.

The current system of antenatal care is acknowledged as being unwieldly and causing some concern to both women and profesionals. However, the Expert group realized that if the number of visits were suddenly reduced then some women would feel anxious. This being so it is suggested that there is greater communication with the women, for example in parentcraft classes or in special drop-in centres in order to explain the rationale of reduced visits and to ally fears.

When considering how information was obtained by women, it was found, not unsurprisingly, that many women received their advice from family and friends.The group suggest that parentcraft classes be tailored to suit the needs of the clients. They heard examples of responses to requests such as grandparent sessions. Purchasers and providers should identify needs, plan in conjunction with the users and review the outcome.

Two other aspects of antenatal care which came under the scrutiny of the Expert Group were screening for fetal abnormalities and antenatal day assessment units. The evidence is that for women the first antenatal visit to hospital often appears rushed and hinged upon the wide range of screening tests available. Within this milieu they are expected to make decisions about the tests they wish to have. The Group saw it as essential that screening tests be associated with sufficient information and proper counselling. Fetal assessment units do not seem to be as yet properly evaluated and although the rationale for them is to reduce the number of antenatal admissions the Group found in the units visited the reduction in admissions was minimal. It would like to see the growth of these units monitored and their effectiveness assessed before new ones are opened.

Place of birth

Professionals providing care for women considered that women would wish to be delivered in hospital and indeed this is what actually happens to 98 per cent of women. However the report found that 72 per cent of women would like to have the choice of a different system of care and delivery.

The alternative to hospital care is delivery in a GP/midwifery led unit or in the home. The safety factor of a home confinement has been hotly debated for decades with no clear answer. The report considers that this being so, it is the duty of the professionals to give the woman as much unbiased and objective information as possible. She will thus be in a position to choose the best option for herself. She must also have time to consider her choice and should have the right to change her mind at whatever stage of her pregnancy she wishes. Non-biased information will, therefore, not only include the hazards of a home confinement but will also give information about the increased possibility of interventions in hospital.

The Report highlights that the 'Domino' scheme and care in the community by a midwife known to the woman is an option which many women find appealing.This being so, it is stated that 'purchasers/providers should consider establishing a midwife led / GP service alongside the specialist facility' (p.2.6.10).

Emergency services

There is often an assumption that the mother is safest in hospital because if an emergency arises expert help will be at hand, whereas help is not so easily available in the community. In reality, this is not always the case as inexperienced doctors may be on duty in the hospital.

The report states that all women having their babies at home should have the availability of efficient and effective back up services in an acute emergency. This being so there should be a well trained and available service with the staff trained to administer intravenous infusion. The professionals who will be present at the birth must have up-to-date training in neonatal resuscitation. Ideally there should be two health professionals present at a home or midwife/GP delivery in order that one is free to resuscitate the baby if needed.

Clear guidelines for neonatal emergencies must be drawn up and midwives working in the community must be supported by general practitioners and by obstetricians 'and that they make clear their readiness to give advice and help if needed'. (Department of Health, 1993a, p. 27).

Care in labour

The primary focus of concern for the professionals should be the woman.Her care should be flexible in order to accommodate her wishes as far as possible. This will be enhanced by the use of a birth plan or other methods of recording the wishes of the woman regarding the birth. The environment should be as supportive and comfortable as possible. The woman should be free to move around in labour and she should be cared for by a midwife whom she knows.

Continuity of care may have the effect of reducing the need for analgesia in labour. However, if the woman wishes to have epidural anaesthesia it is likely to be beneficial if she can meet the anaesthetist for early discussions. Likewise it is useful if there is evidence that the paediatric team will be needed if the woman can meet with them early. 'There should always be clear guidelines for obtaining paediatric support during or following the birth' (Department of Health, 1993a, p. 31).

Postnatal care

The report concerns itself with the care of the mother and baby in the postnatal period and concentrates on the length of stay which is felt should be negotiable as should the provision of advice and support. In the hospital, the midwife should assist the woman to prepare for transfer home, and the woman should be able to contact the midwife when she has returned home.

If the midwife had concerns about the health of the baby she would usually contact the general practitioner in the first instance, but the report addressed the possibility of introducing a system, currently available in some districts, of direct referral to a paediatrician by the midwife. Even when babies or mothers are ill they should be kept together as far as possible and in the case of a multiple birth the siblings should also be kept together. If mothers or babies need to be transferred to specialist units every effort should be made to cater for their need, e.g. in terms of distance or visiting.

Infant feeding is a topic that may make women feel anxious and insecure. They should have the support of a midwife and other professionals who are up-to-date in their knowledge, are supportive, and will listen and give advice and encouragement.

All professionals need to be aware of the possibility of a woman developing postnatal depression and the report supports the view of the Government's document, 'Health of the Nation' that all professional groups will benefit from the development of general and specialist skills in appropriate care and treatment of postnatal depression.

The role of the general practitioner

The report acknowledged that the general practitioner was the professional whose care continued over a long time span and indeed often spanned generations. In general, GPs were very involved in antenatal care but had little involvement with labour. It seems that many GPs are reluctant to refer women to GP/midwife-led units. Midwives were concerned that general practitioners received fees for providing antenatal service which they did not personally provide. The group stated antenatal fees are paid not for undertaking care but 'for ensuring that care is provided' (p.35), and for agreeing to provide intrapartum care should this be required. The Expert Group did not have a remit to review GPs remuneration but did make a recommendation that it is reviewed and also that the obstetric list is reviewed.

There are plans to include maternity services in the list of services that fund-holding general practitioners in pilot projects can purchase. This being so the Group would expect the woman to have a full range of options from which to choose.

The general practitioner is seen to have a valuable role in the provision of continuity of care for women and their families.

The role of the midwife

The report recognizes that women have great confidence in the midwifery profession and talked about the special skills of the midwife and her ability to practice independently. It acknowledges the midwife's role in the management of normal childbirth and the continuing responsibility of the midwife to work with the doctor if matters became complicated.

However, over the past years, fragmentation in delivery of care by midwives has been a consequence of how services were organized. Midwives tended to specialize in one area of care which may have resulted in loss of total care for the woman. In parts of the country team midwifery has been introduced in an attempt to attain greater continuity.

The report gives a brief description of midwifery education. It is now being delivered at a minimum of diploma level and in some areas at degree level. Regardless of the academic level, all midwifery programmes emphasize a balance of clinical and theoretical knowledge and lead to the student becoming competent to practice in both community and hospital before registration as a midwife.

The role of the obstetrician

Some obstetricians would like to spend more time with women who have complicated pregnancies and the group hopes that they will welcome the changes that will enable them to do so. The report considers that overall, the obstetrician will be the main provider of care for women with complications of pregnancy or labour and those that have actual or suspected abnormalities. They will also be more involved in fetal medicine, research, administration and teaching.

It is acknowledged that there may be a group of women who develop complications later in a pregnancy and that the obstetrician, midwife and general practitioner should work as a team to provide the best possible outcome. This may mean also bringing in the skills of the anaesthetists and the paediatrician as early as is practicable. Professional teams are working together to produce protocols and guidelines to care, and in some instances, consumers are also involved in this process, The Group states 'it is this teamwork which ought to be clarified, enhanced and encouraged' (Para.2.12.6).

The role of the obstetric house officer

The report feels that the role of the senior house officer (SHO) should be reviewed with more emphasis placed on the role of learner rather than on service commitments. This will have implications for other professionals. Midwives will have to take on some of the tasks presently the remit of the SHO and consultants will have to spend more time teaching. Experienced midwives may also become more involved in the formal training of the SHO and if so, this will need to be taken account of in staffing levels.

Accessible care

Assessing local needs

The group believes that purchasers and providers should (and some do already) take account of the various needs of local populations. The need of various groups such as the homeless or teenagers should be assessed. It is the purchasers who should secure the particular identified needs of women within service agrements.

Providers should also be able to identify women with particular needs. Standards for care should be agreed with regular audits undertaken to judge how effective they are in achieving consumer satisfaction and the results should be fed back to staff.

It is essential that the service is sensitive to the religious, cultural and linguistic needs of the community it serves and that there are no generalizations about particular groups.

Lay representatives

The report welcomes the views which lay organizations such as the National Childbirth Trust and the Community Health Council currently provide to the maternity service planners. It also supports the view that Maternity Service Liaison Committees (MSLC are maintained and purchasers should ensure that an MSLC with a lay chairperson is established and that the committee's' constitution and remit are agreed.

Communication and information

Poor communication leads to problems and the group feels that purchasers and providers should pay attention to providing good information. Information about services should be published in an agreed form and women should be made aware of the options available to them. This information should be readily available in a range of public places such as post offices and libraries.

Annual figures relating to perinatal care should be published. The increase in community based care will require the development of particular data collection systems.

Uptake of services

Although most women receive antenatal care, there is a wide variation in the degree of acceptability and appropriateness. The evidence from the Maternity Alliance and the National Childbirth Trust shows that many women feel vulnerable when they are pregnant and for some groups a greater degree of vulnerability may be apparant (examples are: the very young, women whose first language is not English and those whose lifestyle may place them outside the mainstream access to the maternity services; the homeless and travellers). Systems which facilitate easy access to the maternity services for those women is seen as an important objective. The MORI survey showed that two per cent of women were not registered with a general practitioner and may therefore have difficulty in obtaining a referral letter when pregnant. The report urged the purchasers and providers to develop a strategy to overcome such problems and ensure that such women are encouraged to have professional care and register with a general practitioner.

Women with disabilities

The report acknowledges that while physical obstructions can cause frustrations for the disabled, prejudice and ignorance on the part of some professionals may be equally vexing. Care should be planned jointly with the women, the midwife, the obstetrician and an appropriate specialist if necessary. Purchasers should ensure that the needs of the disabled are incorporated within service agreements. Disabled women require systems which allow them to easily obtain information regarding the services available as well as facilitating access by improving the design of the facilities which they may use.

Making best use of the services

Access is not just about the first visit. Women informed the Group that even though they attended regularly, they did not feel that they were involved in their care. The Report highlighted Scunthorpe and Medway schemes where antenatal care is given in the home and results in a more relaxed woman who can ask questions more easily. Strategies for better access could include the use of link workers and advocates where necessary The diversity of women who use the maternity services should be portrayed in all promotional material, not only in that which is aimed at particular minority groups. Purchasers should work in close liaison with consumers to monitor the services and to assess whether or not they are accessible to all women.

Education and training

Staff education and training is 'a key element in meeting the diversity of women's needs' (Department of Health, 1993a, p.57). Communication skills, in particular, need improving as part of in service education. Where there are large numbers of women from ethnic groups particular staff training will help staff to be sensitive, non-patronising and above all, sympathetic and kind. The report recognizes that it is a sensitive area but states that ongoing education must be available to ensure staff have the appropriate skills.

Effective and efficient services

Strategic plans

Although there are many local initiatives, the report feels that change is still necessary if the service is to be focussed on women's needs.There has to be an overall strategy for change if the service is to meet the aims specified by purchasers. This being so purchasers should draw up long-term plans and the strategy should contain clear health targets for the next five years and identify how progress will be made. The report particularly encourages the purchasers to look at strategies that are community-based.

Monitoring contracts

Purchasers must monitor the contracts and continue to improve and develop information systems to assess overall needs. They must take into account the views of the women users. This may be done through formal organizations such as the Community Health Councils but purchasers should also seek ways of reaching those who are not normally involved in organizations.

One way may be through consumer surveys, such as that produced by the Office of Population, Censuses and Surveys (Department of Health, 1989)

Research and audit

The Group heard evidence which highlighted the need for new practices to be tested formally. Where there is no proven benefit this fact should be discussed with women. Also there is evidence that some practices such as the use of glycerol impregnated catgut are being continued despite research findings.

The group also support 'the view about the value of audit' (para. 4.3.4.) and in particular welcomes the joint venture between the General Medical Services Committee, the Royal College of General Practitioners and the Royal College of Midwives.

Evaluation of new patterns of care

The report considers that when changes are implemented, they should be evaluated. There are a number of sources of expert advice which can help. These include, amongst others, the National Perinatal Epidemiology Unit in Oxford.

Use of resources

As effectiveness usually goes hand in hand with efficiency, the Group considers that the maternity services are no different from any other area of the NHS in this respect and purchasers should look for ways to maximize efficiency. One of the main ways to do this is to reduce duplication of effort. There is a cost implication in the use of various professional groups who go over the same ground as each other. The implications of duplication as a resource issue must be explored.

The report re-emphasized its concerns about the effectiveness of antenatal care and antenatal day assessment units in particular. It recommends that the Central Research and Development Committee's Standing Group on Health Technology should look at this area.

Action for change

The report identified the three key principles which must underpin effective women-centred care but in order to bring about the change, the cooperation of different groups must be assured. These are: purchasers who will need to review the services and draw up strategic plans; consumers who must be fully involved in the planning and monitoring processes; providers who will need to review their philosophies of care, current practices and organization in order to meet the key principles; clinicians who need to agree guidelines and develop effective teamwork; professional and statutory bodies who need to develop the education and training to meet the needs of the future service and consumer groups who should play an active part in assessing the service on behalf of the women and should work with purchasers and provides in order to bring about change.

Indicators of success
The strategic plans of the providers will need to incorporate standards and a method of monitoring. The report provided ten indicators of success which if achieved will assure that much of what is recommended in the Report will be implemented.

Conclusion

The group hopes that in five years 'the principles embodied in the report will become so widely accepted and its practices so commonplace that 'Changing Childbirth' will have done its work and can take its place on the shelf of history' (Department of Health, 1993a, p.71).

CHAPTER THREE

The Mother as the Focus of Care

'Women want healthy babies and also to be healthy themselves after they have given birth'. (Paragraph 2.1.1)

The issue of safety of mother and baby is not the exclusive prerogative of the professionals.Women too want a safe outcome for themselves and their babies, but they also want to be involved in the decisions made about their care. The onus is upon the providers of care to give sufficient information to the women to enable them to become involved in decisions, a paternalistic attitude is no longer acceptable. The type of care available must be appropriate not just to what is perceived as warranted by the professionals, each woman should believe it is relevant and appropriate to her particular needs. The achievement of this objective will enable not only the spirit of 'Changing Childbirth' to be realized, but the introduction of models of care which are applicable to women during an important period of physical, emotional and social change. These models should include methods of assessing the woman's present physical and emotional health, analysis of the possibility of complications along with appraisal of the physical, social and emotional effects of childbearing to the individual woman and her family. The Expert Maternity Group (Department of Health 1993a) identified that the model of care for childbearing is often more relevant to illness than to a physiological event (p. ii). This may be a result of the influence of the medical profession who are most frequently required to diagnose and treat illness, and where appropriate to give advice to prevent disease and illhealth. The prevalence of the medical model is seen in the scoring systems used to identify pregnancies at risk.

Common to all of the systems is the measurement of risk to the fetus/baby. The parameters most commonly used are premature birth, low birth weight, low Apgar score at birth, or perinatal complications (Alexander and Keirse, 1989). The health outcomes for the woman appear to be forgotten or not considered. Anthropologists and sociologists such as Kitzinger (1989) and Oakley (1993) infer that this is the result of the medicalization of events in women's lives which were previously acknowledged as both social and biological events.

The recognition of childbearing as primarily a non-medical episode requires a shift in emphasis of care. The adoption of the Safe Motherhood Initiative (SMI) as outlined by Maclean (1994) may be one way of achieving a more balanced approach. The aims of the SMI are to enhance the quality and safety of women's lives through the utilization of a combination of health and social strategies, carried out by midwives who are competent and confident to respond to their community. It is in this sphere that all care providers have the greatest challenge, to develop a method of identifying those women whose health and wellbeing may be impaired during pregnancy, labour or the postnatal period, not just their physical and emotional health, but the social implications and effects for the individual woman. It is the social perspective of care which appears to have been forgotten as more medically oriented screening, diagnostic and interventionist techniques have developed (Garcia et al, 1989).

What all women require are systems which provide information to allow them to become part of the decision-making process, and more appropriately to have access to care and support which can assist them through the period of childbearing with minimal physical, emotional or social impairment. While not minimizing the importance of the physical aspects of care, it is within the latter two categories that midwives have their greatest challenge. Garcia et al (1989) point out that 'care givers and medical policy makers ... lack relevant social information about the women for whom they care' (p. 205).

The general practitioner and midwife, working in collaboration, could go some way to addressing this deficit. During the first months of pregnancy the foundation on which care will be based should be established. The traditional methods of collecting a history need to be reviewed. As Rosemary Methvan (1989) pointed out, the design of case notes emphasizes the medical aspects of childbearing to the detriment of social, emotional and behavioural data. Although there have been attempts to implement a more systematic approach to assessing the total needs of women with the introduction of care plans and birth plans, there is no real evidence that social, behavioural and emotional factors receive the same consideration as the medical and obstetrical history. The collection of information on these issues cannot be truly achieved during one interview, therefore an alternative approach is required. One way could be to utilize existing knowledge of the woman's health. The general practitioner will have a total record of the woman's medical history, which contains not just the information normally requested at booking clinic, but minor illness for which medical care was sought. This will give some indication of the general health of the woman, and could be a useful starting point for assessment of the woman's health status and the commencement of specific health education. For example, if a woman has a history of upper respiratory tract infections could a common predisposing factor be identified? Perhaps she is living in poor housing, is under some stress or has an underlying physiological cause. These causes could be explored during early pregnancy. Support and care could then commence.

The quality and accuracy of obtaining specific information on social and emotional factors is dependent upon the willingness of women to disclose such details, and the ability and commitment of professionals to collect the information (Alexander and Keirse, 1989). To expect details which may be very personal on a first encounter is unrealistic, the establishment of a trusting relationship is of the utmost importance. The development of a helping relationship, however, requires more than the appropriate structures to be in place. Each individual midwife needs the skills and knowledge to encourage partnership in care. In studying the midwives' perspectives on the midwife/client relationship, McCrea and Crute (1994) suggest that communication skills need to be well honed in order to overcome any reserve the women may feel, and to overcome any negative or non-responsiveness that may be encountered. This can only be achieved over a period of time. Midwives need to make themselves more accessible to women either by establishing a base where women can get to know them, or by visiting the women at home from an early stage in the pregnancy.

The use of the named midwife as recommended by the Patients' Charter (Department of Health, 1991) would also be beneficial in establishing a reliable association between woman and midwife. It is important, however, that in implementing such a scheme that the named midwife continues care throughout the childbearing period. The Report suggests the introduction of a lead professional who will take the main responsibility for planning and coordinating care. The lead professional may be the midwife, general practitioner or obstetrician, depending upon the needs of the woman, but the choice will ultimately be the woman's. The concept of the lead professional has caused some concern within the ranks of the obstetricians who see its introduction as having,

> 'the potential for isolation of the midwife from contact with general practitioners or obstetricians. Lack of interprofessional communication [is] not thought to be in the best interests of women and their babies' (Dunlop, 1993).

The spirit of 'Changing Childbirth' is that there should be cooperation between all the professionals involved in maternity care. Just as the midwives may approach the medical practitioners for advice and support regarding any medical or obstetric concerns, so too the medical practitioners can utilize the skills of the midwife in the care of women.

One of the important contributions the midwife can offer to the medical practitioners is a knowledge of the social and cultural environment of the woman. This knowledge can help midwives to gain an understanding of the woman's health beliefs and practices and so ensure that information and care is appropriate to the women. For example, the Indian Ayurvedic and Chinese Yin-Yang systems of 'hot' and 'cold' food as a method of maintaining the body's internal balance, irrespective of nutritional values. The classification of foods as 'hot' and 'cold' does not relate to the actual temperature but to the symbolic values associated with certain categories of food. A study of Chinese mothers in London by Tann and Wheeler (cited by Helman, 1990) demonstrated that breast feeding women believed that their diet should be altered in response to the general health of the baby. If the baby had an illness categorised as cold then 'cold' foods which might turn the breast milk cold would be avoided, otherwise the baby's condition might be worsened.

Women's concepts of health also need to be explored. Cornwell (1984) demonstrated that working class women in Bethnall Green saw illness as an unacceptable part of their role and would not, even in the presence of some minor disorders, label themselves as ill. This reluctance was also demonstrated by Pill and Stott (1991) in their study that women identified a 'good mother' as one who 'keeps going' and does not succumb to illness. In exploring the concept of backache Fox (cited by Popay 1992, p. 104) found that those in lower socioeconomic groups considered backache as an unavoidable part of life and therefore not worthy of further investigation. A knowledge of how women locally perceive their health is important to enable health professionals to ask the right questions to assess women's health status, and begin to appraise the needs of the individual.

An awareness of local employment patterns for women may also be significant in assessing risk to the pregnancy. Namelle and Laumon (1984) found that working conditions can influence the pregnancy outcome; preterm births are associated with a long working week, standing during work, having few breaks and having a job which is especially tiring. Oakley (1993) proposes that these conditions could be pertinent to many women who do not go out to work but bear the main burden of caring for the home and other children. Giving information to women on how to care for themselves requires a knowledge of any special facilities or benefits that may be on offer within the place of employment (Garcia et al, 1989) or available within the community, such as play schemes for children. Where appropriate, extra support and care can be planned. Oakley (1992) found that where social support was given by midwives there were fewer lower birthweight babies, less antenatal admissions to hospital, more spontaneous onset of labour and spontaneous vaginal deliveries. Both mothers and babies were found to be healthier at six weeks and one year after the birth. Women's perceptions of the value of the care remained positive one year after delivery.

Once the midwife has the appropriate knowledge of the social and cultural environment she can begin to build an understanding of the context in which women may make decisions regarding their care and can give appropriate information and support to encourage them to make informed choices.

In making choices women require information on the alternatives available and the consequences of their choice. This information should not only be on the risks of rejecting one particular form of care, but the effects of accepting care offered. Heelas and Morris (1992) suggest that the enterprise culture has entered the professional territories. This has the effect of expecting people to exercise their freedom of choice as 'enterprising consumers', but in order to choose responsibly one must know what is being offered (Strathern, 1992) and choice is often not an option because of lack of knowledge (Stacey, 1976). Although the obligation for ensuring information is available for women rests with all the providers of care, the midwife may need to take the lead in this role in order to function within the professional role identified by the United Kingdom Central Council for Nursing, Midwifery and Health Visiting. The Code of Professional Conduct states:

> In the exercise of your professional accountability, [you] must act always in such a manner as to promote and safeguard the interests and well-being of patients and clients and ensure that no action or omission on your part, or within your sphere of responsibility, is detrimental to the interests, condition or safety of patients and clients (UKCC, 1992).

When working to this Code midwives should reflect on the information given to women regarding the type of antenatal care, the place of delivery and the pattern of postnatal care available. It is now accepted that traditional shared care is no longer an efficient and effective way of ensuring the diagnosis of deviations from normal or in ensuring that individual needs of women are met.(Hall et al 1980) The Expert Group (Department of Health 1993a) acknowledged that despite the evidence there has been little change in the pattern of antenatal care (p. 20). The midwife is in the position to give information to women and allow them to make the decision on whether or not they continue with the customary care or opt for some other form. An alternative must be discussed and an acceptable pattern of antenatal care established.

In discussing the place of delivery do midwives give unbiased information regarding the comparative risks of home and hospital delivery? If a woman with perceived risk requests a home delivery it is usual for the professionals to point out the risks and seek to persuade the women to book for a hospital confinement, but if a woman with an uncomplicated pregnancy requests a hospital confinement no such information on the risks of hospital care are explained. The Health Committee Second Report (House of Commons 1992) reminds us 'that the policy of encouraging all women to give birth in hospitals cannot be justified on grounds of safety', and there is some evidence to suggest that women with normal uncomplicated pregnancies actually fare less well in hospital in terms of both morbidity and mortality (Tew, 1990, Klein et al 1983, Campbell and Macfarlane 1987). Women are often cajoled into having their babies in hospital because the professionals tell them it is safer and women do want to do what is best for their babies even if this means that their own needs are secondary. Making the woman central to care means that their needs should also be considered. Midwives should be aware of the potential for undermining the status of women or making them 'invisible'within the system of care. Analysing the views of women and men regarding ultrasound, Sandelowski (1994) found that while it enhances the experience of women by allowing them to share their pregnancy with their partners, there is the risk that the women and their experiences are seen as peripheral by making 'seeing and getting a picture of the fetus at least as significant as carrying the fetus' Sandelowski also discovered that women's knowledge of their fetus and pregnancy was rejected in favour of the knowledge gained through ultrasound. The Expert Group reiterates that the woman should be central to all care, so the challenge for midwives is to ensure that women's views and experiences receive equal recognition as technological findings.

During labour the prospect for obscurity is greater. The use of techniques of intervention along with machinery to manipulate and control labour reduces the uterus to a machine capable of being manipulated and the woman to the role of labourer. The fetus becomes the important end product and the rights of the woman as an individual are diminished (Martin 1987). But it is not only the use of technology which excludes the women. Kirkham (1989) found that the actions of midwives and their use of language had a profound effect on the treatment of women during labour. The use of phrases such as 'dear' and 'lovey' had the effect of infantalising women and thereby making them vulnerable and powerless within the care setting. Once in this situation women feel unable to assert their wishes regarding the management of their care. Kirkham also found that focussing attention on monitors or other machines by the midwife barred the woman from any encounter with the midwife. All these factors reduce the status of women, render them passive objects in the process of production and powerless to do anything about it. A shift in the focus of care is required in order to ensure that women become the main focal point and they are empowered to contribute to the overall plan of care.

It is often believed that the postnatal period is when the midwife and woman can establish a truly equal partnership. In the main postnatal care is the domain of the midwife, especially when the woman returns home. The introduction of selective postnatal visiting in the home appears to have been accepted as part of standard practice. The United Kingdom Central Council for Nursing, Midwifery and Health Visiting (UKCC), have seen fit to make a statement regarding selective visiting by stating:

> 'Each midwife is personally responsible and accountable for the exercise of professional judgment and determining appropriate practice in relation to mother and baby. This, naturally, includes judgments about the number of visits and any additional visits required in the postnatal period. The range of midwifery care, including timing of visits, should be discussed with the mother.' (Registrars Letter 11/1992)

The importance of discussion on the pattern of postnatal care in relation to the needs of the individual woman is not easily identifiable,midwives generally make the decisions regarding the number and timing of visits, and the decision is usually related to the work load of the particular midwife (Hamilton,1994). The main feature of postnatal visits appears to be the physical well being of the baby and woman (Marsh and Sargent,1991), with the baby being the major consideration (Hamilton,1994). The status of women is again secondary and their power to make decisions is eroded. As Oakley (1993) points out 'the single most difficult aspect of motherhood today is that other people are always telling mothers what they ought to do.' (p.100) When this advice is not congruent with their own experience and expectations it has the effect of alienating women from the whole health system. It should not be surprising if women fail to take the advice which is not requested or not perceived as relevant.

Much is said about the importance of empowering women to take control and make decisions regarding their care.Empowerment helps to facilitate decision making by improving the individuals self-concept and by enhancing self-esteem, but in order to be empowered women require awareness,information and assertiveness (Patterson and Burns,1990).

For the midwife this means raising the women's awareness that they are capable of making decisions,giving them the knowledge required to make the decision, respecting the decision made and ensuring that others also honour the decision.This may be contrary to some midwives' beliefs and practices, they may feel that women will not make the 'right' decisions but this implies that women do not want a healthy outcome to their pregnancy and there is no evidence to support this belief.

In reviewing the literature relating to compliance with treatment in diabetic women Patterson and Burns (1990) point out that education alone is not effective in increasing compliance but where the women were taught basic assertiveness skills not only did they have a more positive approach to the management of their condition,they were more confident in their ability to manage their condition and to seek help when necessary. Applying these principles to antenatal care, it may be possible to encourage women to take responsibility for the number of antenatal visits required by educating them on symptoms which require further investigation, such as backache, headaches, visual disturbances or oedema. It would also be possible to supply women with equipment with which to test their urine.

While it may not be practical for midwives to conduct formal assertiveness training for all women, it is within their role to educate women and it may be appropriate to include some aspects such as, how to ask for information or choices available and the possible consequences of choice within parentcraft classes rather than some of the topics presently included. But this will not ensure that the most vulnerable women are helped as they are least likely to actually attend such classes. The midwife must find alternatives for these women. Schott (1994) suggests that listening to these women instead of undertaking routine checks which have little proven benefit would be a start. By listening in an empathetic way the midwife may find that the women can indeed find their own solutions to problems, but if not then listening may give the midwife greater insight into the problems of the women and better equip the midwife to offer information which is appropriate to the individual woman's situation. This will encourage more relevant decision making and may also have the effect of increasing the woman's self-esteem. If greater self-esteem and self-concept could be achieved by those women who normally have least control over their lives during what is acknowledged as an important social and biological event for all women then midwives would truly be 'with woman'. In the words of Schott (1994),

> 'Let's not leave any woman holding her baby without having conveyed to her our complete respect and belief in her ability to think clearly, to make decisions and to be a good parent.'

CHAPTER FOUR

Challenges to the Medical Practitioners

For general practitioners and obstetricians the 'Changing Childbirth' Report (Department of Health, 1993a) offers unprecedented challenges – the opportunity to deliver their expert skills in the most flexible and appropriate manner to ensure that women who need or require their skills have access to them. The skill of the obstetrician is in the care of those women whose health is likely to be impaired by childbearing, where complications arise during the pregnancy, labour or puerperium or where the fetus is at risk. The complementary roles of all professionals involved in maternity care requires them to work in a cooperative way to ensure that women, whatever their risk status, receive care which respects their needs and wishes.

The general practitioner, who presently is the most common primary contact for women who want access to the maternity services, has a major responsibility for ensuring that women are made aware of the services available and how they may access them. This role requires a knowledge of the physical, social and emotional perspective of each woman. The general practitioner will usually have this information and can use it as a basis for discussion with the woman so that she is helped to understand the patterns of care available and make an informed decision on the best care for her individual circumstances.

It is feasible that the woman may want professional advice on the risks to her and her baby before she makes any decision regarding care. This is easily given to those women who have existing medical conditions which pregnancy can complicate or which can be hazardous to the health of the woman or fetus. Predicting complications by the use of elaborate risk scoring techniques is less accurate (Alexander and Keirse, 1989). The disadvantages of using risk scoring systems which are not proven to be of benefit are described by Stirrat (1988) as 'myths' related to obstetric care. These are:

'If a factor causes a catastrophic event ... in some women, then there will inevitably be others in whom the same factor causes lesser degrees of harm.'

'A test which has been proven to be of benefit to women or fetuses at high risk or disease, is of benefit to all regardless of risk' (pp. 82–84).

If these beliefs are translated into care there is a danger that women will be subjected to treatments and interventions which have not been established to be of benefit and whose hazards are unknown (Alexander and Keirse, 1989). There is also the issue of the cost of unproven therapies. Given the finite resources of the National Health Service, it is important that resources both human and monetary are effectively and efficiently utilized.

For the woman, the danger is that they are more likely that to be categorized into a risk group and the emphasis will be on finding something wrong rather than finding something right. Many of the 'problems' found are referred to the obstetrician who takes over responsibility for care (Oakley and Houd, 1990). As a result there is increased possibility that women's choice is minimized or totally excluded.

Systems need to be developed which are flexible enough to allow the most appropriate professional to take the lead in care at any time during the childbearing period in response to the changing health status of the woman or fetus. It would be feasible to treat a woman presenting for the first time with an uncomplicated pregnancy as suitable for care in the community by either the general practitioner or midwife. Even in the presence of social factors which are known to increase the risk of complications, e.g. poor housing and poverty, it may be more appropriate to at least commence care with one of the primary carers as the lead professional. This approach may even be beneficial for these women, as it will allow the midwife or general practitioner to establish a relationship with the women and work with them to identify their individual needs or anxieties. Health promotion and support can commence early in pregnancy. Oakley (1992) found increased social support by a midwife actually benefited the woman and fetus/baby, in that their physically and psychological wellbeing was significantly improved. If deviations from normal occur then transfer of lead professional to the obstetrician could be arranged.

It is the concept of lead professional that seems to cause the greatest discord between the professions. Dunlop (1993) writing in his capacity as the Honorary Secretary of the Royal College of Obstetricians and Gynaecologists states,

> 'It was felt that this term [lead professional] would encourage the idea of ownership of a pregnancy by one professional to the exclusion of others and was therefore potentially divisive.'

This statement appears to imply that professionals cannot cooperate and work together for the benefit of the woman and her pregnancy. To have a named obstetrician, general practitioner or midwife as the person who will be responsible for the majority of care, and to see that person regularly during pregnancy, when in labour and post-delivery will give women the continuity of care which they desire.

The woman should know that the lead professional will be the person who has the greatest understanding of her individual needs and wishes and is the best person to give her any advice or information she requires regarding her condition. This does not exclude other professionals from giving care, but it may prevent conflicting advice if others involved in care acknowledge the important role of the lead professional and agree to take a supportive role, contributing their unique skills to the good of the woman. The 'Changing Childbirth' Report (Department of Health, 1993a) states that the women should 'feel confident that the professionals are working in harmony, as a team, supporting her and her family with clear patterns of referral and a smooth transfer of information and responsibility' (p.6). This does not imply that referral should always be one way.

There is no reason why consultants cannot advise women with uncomplicated pregnancies that the general practitioner or midwife is more appropriate as the lead professional, just as the general practitioner or midwife advise a woman whose pregnancy becomes complicated that consultant care is more appropriate. Referral back to the midwife or general practitioner may also be applicable in those instances where obstetric opinion is required but no abnormality is diagnosed. For example, in a case of suspected fetal growth retardation where the opinion of the obstetrician is requested and investigations demonstrate that fetal growth is within normal limits, then the women could be redirected back to the primary carer(s).

Establishing care within the community can also help those women who often fail to gain the best from the systems available. These include women from black and ethnic minorities, the disabled, travellers, the very young and those in poor social circumstances. The establishment of midwifery teams with a named midwife could help to break down the barriers which exist between the professionals and these groups, particularly if the midwife develops her knowledge of the individual circumstances and can offer the help and information required by liaising with local groups or significant individuals within the community. Once a pattern of care is established with the woman she too can be given appropriate information to allow her to make a choice regarding subsequent care. If specialist obstetric care is required and the lead professional changes, the woman can be reassured that the named midwife or her general practitioner will not relinquish all responsibility, but will continue care under the direction of the obstetrician.

Cooperation between professionals is essential especially in situations where low risk women choose the obstetrician as the lead professional, or women with complicated pregnancies opt for midwifery or general practitioner led care. When women choose it should not be seen as a rejection of one professional in favour of another, but rather the woman opting for the care which she sees as most appropriate.

It is in the provision of primary care that coordination and cooperation is particularly important. The move to community care could result in an overload of the primary care providers, particularly midwives and general practitioners. To facilitate the perceived increase in community care, additional resources will be required. This can be achieved by the introduction of team midwifery with previously hospital-based midwives undertaking community care. Financial implications will need to be considered by the purchasers (see Chapter 7). Patterns of care will also need to be reviewed. The continuing use of the present model of antenatal care which has no proven benefit may mean that other areas of care are neglected, in particular postnatal care. The Expert Group recommend that the structure of antenatal care is reviewed and the proposals of the Royal College of Obstetricians and Gynaecologists (RCOG, 1982) be implemented and evaluated.

For the general practitioner and midwife, as the first contacts for the pregnant woman and the last association at the end of the childbearing period, the process of evaluation could be a collaborative affair. They have all the necessary information to allow analysis of the outcomes of care. Locally collected statistics and measured outcomes could become an integral part of their overall assessment of standards of care. For example, if a woman does develop a complication they could examine whether or not there were any contributory factors which could have been identified. The general practitioner and midwife could also collaborate on the setting and monitoring of standards, this would ensure that evaluation would be an ongoing process and would contribute to establishing a more responsive team able to provide care which is meaningful to the women. Collaboration may also enhance the professional relationship as each recognizes their complementary roles in the provision of care, whether this be antenatal, intranatal or postnatal care.

While the provision of community antenatal care may not cause great controversy, the suggestion of choice for home births has been the basis for much discussion. The RCOG have stated 'that this (home confinement) is not a safe alternative to delivery in properly equipped surroundings.' (RCOG, 1993). Regardless of the views of the professionals, the fact remains that women do have the right to opt for a home confinement. The Expert Group (Department of Health,1993a) acknowledge much of the discussion regarding choice was focused upon the place of birth but 'believe that home confinement may have come to symbolize "real" choice because of the more personalized service that it offers and the fact that it explicitly leaves control in the hands of the woman and her family' (p.99). The choice does not need to be so limited, as there are many alternatives to consultant led hospital delivery. The domino system could be more widely utilized and the introduction of midwifery led beds within the consultant unit could be a feasible alternative for those women who feel more secure by being nearer to all the specialist services should these be required. In some areas there are also general practitioner/midwifery units available but a reluctance to use such units was acknowledged by the Expert Group.

It may be pertinent to review how such units can be used for the benefit of women who do not wish the high-tech environment of the district general hospital, but do not wish to give birth at home. The aim could be to create an environment which is relaxing, conducive to encouraging women to remain mobile during labour and which supports the adoption of alternative positions for delivery. Care during labour and delivery can be delivered by members of the midwifery team with general practitioner involvement. These units could also be used for the training of future general practitioners. It would give them opportunity to gain experience and confidence in the care of normal labours and deliveries and may help them to see childbearing not as a risk laden event but rather a physiological process, which in the main progresses free of complications. Having had this experience future general practitioners may be more confident to offer community based care.

The use of these alternatives for women with uncomplicated pregnancies means that the midwife or general practitioner as the lead professional will take responsibility for a large proportion of women leaving the obstetrician free to devote time and expertise to women who present with or develop complications. Obstetricians can be free to develop their expertise in the conditions which complicate childbearing and develop further the strategies to deal with such conditions. Time can be used to explain to women the reasons for medical interventions, and the possible outcomes of care. Cooperation with other experts can help improve the overall outcomes. Involvement of anaesthetists for those women who may need operative intervention can enhance the women's understanding of the alternatives and allow her to make the most appropriate choice for anaesthesia.

Paediatric skill will also be imperative where it is known in advance that the baby will require intensive care. Discussion with the parents in advance with a visit to the neonatal unit can help alleviate the fear which parents may feel. It must not be forgotten that the midwife will also have a role in the support and care of this category of women. The named midwife can work closely with the obstetrician and other experts to help the woman understand the reasons for intervention and to give the social and psychological support required to minimize the anxiety which the woman may feel. Helping the woman to become involved in ensuring a safe and satisfying outcome would be important, but the support and care of women where a satisfactory outcome is not anticipated or achieved is crucial. Where a baby is stillborn or dies soon after birth the support of the named midwife can continue after the woman has left the hospital. This continuity may go some way to helping the family to come to terms with the loss of their baby.

In providing postnatal care to all women, good communication between the professionals is important, and the level of cooperation developed during the antenatal and intranatal periods can be crucial in ensuring that care is continuous. Whatever type of care chosen, women will return home to the care of the general practitioner and midwife so they will require a knowledge of events during pregnancy and delivery. Where the obstetrician undertook the role of lead professional and the named midwife worked with the obstetrician in the delivery of care, continuity is more likely. The midwife can also ensure that the general practitioner has the knowledge required to be involved in the care postnatally.

Continuity of care into the postnatal period can help with the diagnosis and management of postnatal depression. The midwife or general practitioner with their knowledge of the woman can gauge any changes in behaviour which may occur. Early intervention can be initiated. This may be extra support from the midwife or general practitioner for those suffering from postnatal blues or the opinion and treatment by the psychiatrist and care by the community psychiatric nurse in more serious cases.

The importance of cooperation and communication between all professionals involved in the care of women during the process of childbearing is a consistent feature of the report. The overriding principle is that women should have care which is safe, satisfying, respects their wishes and treats them as individuals capable of making decisions in their own and their baby's interest. All professionals have a duty to respond to these wishes by offering their expert skills to the women. The women should decide who is the most appropriate lead professional, but be reassured that this can always change should the need arise.

CHAPTER FIVE

Maternity Service Provision

'Change will not happen *to* you or *for* you: it will be you who make it happen' (Lesley Page, 1994)

Implementation of the recommendations of 'Changing Childbirth' (Department of Health, 1993a) inevitably mean changes in the provision and organization of midwifery care. Midwives, both practitioners and managers should be anxious to be involved in the process. Managers will be required to drive the changes and practitioners will be required to alter not just their methods of delivery of care but their whole philosophy of care. Midwives can view this as a challenge to shake off the shackles of the last 20 years and use the opportunity to develop further the service into one which women have indicated they want. If midwives do not meet the challenge and grasp the opportunities they could become obstetric nurses.

What is certain is that the delivery of maternity care will change, but in what way is dependent upon midwives themselves and how they face the challenge. In particular, midwives who are responsible for day-to-day contact with women and their families must be willing to evaluate their present methods of delivering care, to consider what changes are required and how these may be best implemented. Managers will be required to support and encourage midwives to critically appraise practice and help them to find ways to implement the changes. Supervisors of Midwives will also have an important role in enabling and supporting midwives through the changes required.

The NHS Management Letter EL(93)72 (Department of Health, 1993c) has identified indicators of success which are to be achieved within five years. The indicators which are particularly pertinent to midwifery practice are that:

- Every woman should know one midwife who ensures continuity of her midwifery care: the named midwife.
- At least 30 per cent of women should have the midwife as the named professional.
- At least 75 per cent of women delivered in a maternity unit should know the person who cares for them during labour.
- Midwives should have direct access to some midwifery beds in all maternity units.
- At least 30 per cent of women delivered in a maternity unit should be admitted under the management of the midwife.

The most obvious interpretation is that continuity of care is essential in the delivery of midwifery care, but underpinning the philosophy is that continuity of carer should also be considered. There is a fundamental difference in these two concepts and how they influence the organization of care. It may be pertinent to reflect upon these two perspectives, their similarities and differences, and how they affect the care which women receive.

Continuity of care

Continuity of care relates to the care that the women receive, it should be consistent, reliable and non-conflicting. Women should not be in the position of having different professionals giving incongruous information leaving them confused as who they should believe. Treating the woman as the focus of care with unique individual needs was described by Murphy-Black (1992) as continuity of caring. But whatever the name (care or caring) coordination is essential. The implementation of the 'named midwife' scheme for each woman presenting for care would be a useful starting point. The named midwife would be responsible for undertaking the booking interview and commencing records. At this time women could receive information regarding options for care with a later meeting to discuss choices and record the woman's wishes. Periodic review throughout the childbearing period by the lead professional would be essential to allow reassessment and update of choices and to evaluate how options and choices are implemented. Recording clearly and concisely the woman's wishes and the plan of care is essential and these records should be available to every professional who is involved in care. Encouraging women to carry their own complete set of records is one way of ensuring that all involved in care have a comprehensive knowledge of the woman's wishes and an unabridged version of the care given. For women with complicated pregnancies who require obstetric care, the named midwife may be particularly desirable to support and assist her during what may be a particularly stressful period, but it is important that the facility should be available to all women especially where a number of professionals share care. The named midwife can act as the agent of continuity of care.

While acknowledging that continuity of care can be difficult to achieve if a large number of midwives or other professionals are involved in the care process, it may be more pertinent to reflect on the words of the Expert Group:

> 'Services can be reorganized, roles and responsibilities altered, but we are convinced that the most fundamental change that needs to occur is one of attitude on the part of some care-givers' (p.12).

The attitude change required to achieve continuity of care is one where all midwives are willing to acknowledge the named midwife's responsibility for coordination of care and their own role in ensuring that care planned is implemented in a spirit of cooperation and support. How often has the opposite occurred? Who would disagree with Flint (1993) when she says 'relationships (between midwives) are often quite strained... It is impossible for a midwife to ask a more senior midwife about a mistake she thinks she might have made because the midwife knows that she will be castigated, or gossiped about or even disciplined.' (p.8)

Linking this thought to continuity of care, can the named midwife be sure that others will follow to the best of their ability the care planned in conjunction with the woman? In some instances the answer may be yes, but unless all midwives start supporting and cooperating with each other and accept that others' methods of delivering care can be as competent as theirs, the answer will be no, and the introduction of any scheme to ensure continuity of care will be doomed to failure.

Continuity of care also requires cooperation between all the professionals involved in care. Consistency of approach can be facilitated by the development of agreed policies and protocols, particularly in the care of women who have or develop complications, and in the management of emergency situations. The involvement of the anaesthetist and paediatrician as well as other professionals who may form part of the multidisciplinary team is essential so that each professional may contribute his or her expertise. Merely formulating policies and protocols will not ensure that care is consistent, this requires a willingness on the part of all professionals to carry out the agreed procedures. Regular review is essential to assess compliance and effectiveness and to update management prescribed in the light of new knowledge. Using the policies and protocols will ensure that in the absence of the lead professional, women can be reassured that care recommended is compatible to that which their lead professional would suggest.

In their evidence to the Expert Group women indicated that what they wanted was a known midwife to care for them during labour. Perhaps what they want is for the person who cares for them to treat them as individuals capable of discussing and earnestly considering their wishes for care during labour. It may be that this is more likely to occur within the present system of care if the midwife is known to the woman prior to labour and will be around after the delivery. If the same midwife has to care for a women following delivery it is probable that she is more likely to adhere to a plan of care than the midwife who has never met the woman before labour and may never meet the woman again.

The challenge for the managers of the profession is to create an environment which fosters unity and harmony. It will mean encouraging and supporting those midwives who want to implement continuity of care and cajoling those who are less willing to accept the philosophy. It also requires managers who are willing to undertake regular audit to ensure that care planned with the women is consistent with their wishes and that the plan is implemented to the satisfaction of the women. Areas for improvement can be identified and targets established to ensure that standards are maintained. It may also be possible to identify areas where development of staff may be needed in order to improve the service offered.

The introduction of the named midwife will require some adjustment to the method of delivery of care. The Report suggests that 'wherever possible the named midwife should be located in the community.

This neighbourhood midwife should feel comfortable practising both in the community and hospital.' (p.14) The implication is that for a large proportion of women, midwifery care should be undertaken by community-based midwives. To achieve a target of 75 per cent of women delivering in a maternity unit having care by a midwife known to them may initially appear somewhat daunting, but this figure could be worked towards by perhaps initially placing a target of 30 per cent. This figure is not unattainable for most units. Take, for instance, a unit which has 3,000 deliveries per year, it is possible that 1,000 could be guaranteed a known midwife by some reorganization of the system, and by increasing the availability of the Domino system. Different approaches have been attempted, mainly a reorganization of midwives into groups or teams, with varying degrees of success (Institute of Manpower Studies, 1993). It is not intended to detail all of these schemes but many did not achieve the goal of increasing continuity. This does not mean that in another place they may not work, it requires commitment to change long-standing working practices on the part of midwives to make it work.

The problems of introducing continuity of care without some degree of continuity of carer is apparent in the evidence produced by many of the schemes implemented. It may be that schemes to introduce continuity of carer should be the goal.

Continuity of carer

Continuity of carer implies that total care is given by a specific midwife, but it is doubtful that this ideal can be achieved for every woman, so workable alternatives have been sought. In many places team midwifery has been established as a means of working towards continuity of carer. The Institute of Manpower Studies (1993) compiled a survey of the status of team midwifery within the United Kingdom. Three main models of team midwifery were identified: those providing hospital care only; those providing community care only; and teams providing care in both community and hospital. The model which most successfully achieved integrated care was the one which consisted of both community and hospital midwives. The survey also found large variations in what constituted a 'team', some teams had as many as 23 midwives, but the average was between 11 and 13 per team. Not surprisingly caseloads, when these were defined, tended to be large and many women did not have a known midwife care for her during labour. Continuity of carer was not being achieved.

It must be acknowledged that these first attempts at alternative organization of care formed a basis on which more appropriate systems could be established. As detailed by Ward and Frohlich (1994) midwifery services in Bristol introduced their scheme in 1991. A team of six midwives undertook a caseload of 300 women per year based within three general practitioner surgeries. Problems were identified and solutions sought. At first all six midwives undertook care in all three surgeries, but in order to achieve the 'named midwife' the caseload was further divided. Two midwives are allocated to each of the three surgeries to give antenatal and postnatal care to the women who are registered at the surgery, other members of the team are introduced at parentcraft sessions or on home visits. This ensures that women have a named midwife who is responsible for care but that when in labour the woman can be guaranteed a familiar face. Care of complicated pregnancies and labours including caesarean sections is also undertaken by members of the team. Because only one team is in operation it is not possible for the team to undertake all care for all their defined caseload because of the demands upon their time. Team members do not undertake care for women who are admitted to the antenatal ward, although they do become involved when either induction of labour is arranged or when the woman is discharged home. The provision of postnatal care in hospital is undertaken by hospital based midwives. Similar problems following the introduction of just one team were also experienced by midwives in Oxford (Bower, 1993). It may be that these problems can be overcome if more than one team is introduced or if midwives within the postnatal areas link with different teams and get to know the women before they are admitted to their wards. Midwives in one of the teams in Rhondda have implemented a similar scheme. They have linked with two hospital-based midwives, one on night duty and the other on day duty. When one of these midwives is on duty the team midwife does not come to the hospital, care is undertaken by the link midwife (Flint,1993).

Other team schemes have been introduced, these include the identification of a caseload for each individual midwife. Partnerships are created by pairing-up two midwives and further support by defining a group practice of six midwives (Page et al, 1994). This scheme has not yet been evaluated. The South East London Midwifery Group Practice is a group of self-employed midwives who have secured, initially for six months, an NHS contract to deliver midwifery care. They have chosen to reserve 75 per cent of bookings for women who have particular socioeconomic factors in their lives which may place them 'at risk'. Fourteen categories have been identified which range from specific social factors such as poor housing and poverty status to more specific health problems such as women who are HIV positive, or have mental health difficulties (Demilew, 1994). Again evaluation of this scheme is awaited.

These attempts at implementing a team approach to care have identified issues which need to be considered. Introducing one or two teams within the total service does not significantly decrease the work load of midwives giving traditional care. Within the labour ward where midwives may be responsible for the care of two or three women, it may appear that their team colleagues have less demands made upon them as they care for just one woman. The same issue can arise within the postnatal areas. Managers need to be sensitive to these factors and ensure that all midwives are sufficiently supported and informed regarding possible effects on them. Before teams are introduced throughout the area, the need for core staff within the hospital must be considered. Ball et al (1992) have suggested that the role of midwives within the delivery suite would be to provide care for women who require obstetrician led care. They would give support to team midwives, develop specialist skills in the care of complicated labours and care of sick women and babies, and also have a role in teaching specialist skills to junior midwives and junior medical staff. Midwives within the ward areas would also develop skills in the care of women who develop complications during pregnancy and the postnatal period. Their skills would complement the skills of the team midwives and ensure that women would receive the care of a midwife whatever her circumstances.

For many midwives the concept of team midwifery may cause considerable anxiety as they consider the effect on their personal lives. Stock (1993) acknowledges that although a small team does result in more continuity of care for women, the midwives must be prepared to radically change their existing working patterns with longer shift and continuing responsibility outside 'normal' working hours. Many midwives have family commitments, either children or elderly parents for whom arrangements will have to be made. If hours are irregular then any such arrangements may be difficult to achieve, and may cause a great deal of stress to the midwives. This will inevitably affect the quality of care offered to women.

The challenge for the managers is to ensure that a woman-centred service is delivered by midwives who are not constantly trying to balance the demands of the job with the demands of home. But midwives should not always expect their managers or others to find solutions to their problems. As professionals offering a service it is they who should be exploring and discussing options which allow them to use their expertise and skills to deliver that service. A flexible work-share system between two midwives within a team may be one answer but there may be solutions other than the team approach to care. The recommendations of Ball et al (1992) could also be considered. They suggest the use of a system of primary and associate midwives. The planning and delivery of care to a defined caseload would be the responsibility of the primary midwife with associate midwives contributing to the care to provide a complete 24-hour service.

For managers the issue of clinical grading requires major consideration as the current grading criteria may actually restrict the professional role of midwives at the lower grades. For example, it could be perceived that a midwife within the E grade band could not take responsibility for a caseload of women, but what has not been considered is that E grade midwife may have many years experience but is confined within a role perhaps because she can only work part-time. Managers need to explore the possibility that restricting the practice midwives in this or other ways within the confines of the clinical grading prevents midwives fulfilling the role of the midwife as defined by the Code of Practice which states:

> 'she must be able to give the necessary supervision, care and advice to women during pregnancy, labour and postpartum period, to conduct deliveries on her how responsibility and to care for the newborn and infant. This care includes preventative measures, the detection of abnormal conditions in mother and child, the procurement of medical assistance and the execution of emergency measures in the absence of medical help' (UKCC 1994).

It appears that continuity of carer and the implementation of team midwifery could be impeded by the present structure, but managers may be confronted by such problems without the possibility of implementing the career structure recommended by Ball et al (1992) especially if the structure had increased cost implications. Alternatives may need to be considered. If the main objective is that the woman must be the focus of care, based on her identified needs and carried out in consultation with her, there is no reason to believe that this can only be achieved by a team approach. Charles (1993) warns that an obsession to achieve this goal may discourage any attempt at other forms of achieving improvements in care.

Implementing continuity of carer does not automatically mean that the quality of care is enhanced. Lee (1994) in her study of the value and meaning of elements of care provided by a team of community midwives found that the women first wanted a midwife who inspires confidence and trust, and secondly one who is a safe and competent practitioner. Having a known midwife was placed fifth by the women. The mean ranking of the ideal elements of care placed the bleep system of contacting the midwife as the most important with knowing the midwife who undertakes care in labour as next most important. Lee concludes, 'although the possibility of good care is enhanced if a midwife knows the women she attends, continuity of carer may not be essential for giving and receiving good quality care.'

Assessing the quality of care

Before any change can be implemented it is important that an evaluation of existing care is undertaken. This can be achieved in two ways: an appraisal of personal practice or a more extensive audit of the provision of total midwifery care. For critical assessment of personal practice midwives could work together, for example, a group of community midwives may wish to examine how they currently operate the named midwife scheme, or how information regarding choices is offered to women. Using the examples outlined in 'The Survey of Good Communications Practice in Maternity Services' (Department of Health, 1993a) could give midwives a basis on which to assess the service they offer.

In Staffordshire, a general practitioner and midwife offer weekly informal group discussions for women with time allocated to those who wish to talk privately to either professional. Quality of care is also monitored by follow-up questionnaire. An antenatal drop-in clinic is provided in Redhill, Surrey along with a telephone link which women can call any time they have a query regarding their pregnancy. Salford midwives provide a user-friendly pregnancy club for pregnant teenagers, while in Hamilton, Scotland a Maternity Roadshow of display boards which are transported throughout the community give information to women regarding the choices available to them regarding their care. These and the many more examples offer midwives a foundation for the assessment of their practice. Comparison can be made between what is currently offered locally and the services provided in other parts of the country.

It is important that the opinion of local women regarding what they want from the midwifery services, is taken into consideration. This requires a more extensive evaluation coordinated on a district basis. The OPCS survey manual, 'Women's Experience of Maternity Care' (Department of Health, 1989) is a tried and tested method of assessing women's views of the maternity care. Mid-Staffordshire have used this approach and identified areas where care could be improved. These included:

- the need for women to be given more information regarding type and place of delivery
- increased knowledge of topics related to labour
- more time to talk to staff throughout the period of care. (Wardle, 1994)

Using the same survey in Redbridge, Brooks and Black (1994) found that women wanted the following:

- Antenatal services close to home
- Full involvement in care plans and decisions
- Continuity of care, choice of lead professional
- Equal and respectful partnership
- Appointments which are accurate and individual
- Information which is comprehensive and clear
- Open access to a trusted, familiar community midwife
- Personal care, advice and support.

It may be that the requirements of women in different parts of the country vary, so it is important that their views are sought prior to implementation of any changes, not just their opinion on services currently provided but a more comprehensive assessment of their wishes. Women from minority groups or those with special needs may require particular consideration. Garcia et al (1989) remind us 'that women at the margins do not have confidence in the services e.g. the young, unmarried, grande multiparae and the poor'.

What must be remembered is that the Department of Health has not dictated the schemes of care which are essential to ensure that the indicators are met, although it was acknowledged that the successful introduction of team midwifery can go some considerable way to meet the objectives. It is not only continuity of care or carer that needs to be considered by the midwifery profession, two other issues need to be addressed: the introduction of midwifery led beds and a possible increase in demand for home births.

Home births

Presently in this country 98 per cent of women give birth in a consultant hospital unit, but 72 per cent indicate that they would like to have the chance to consider an alternative system. Of those who would like a choice 22 per cent expressed a wish to have the option of a home delivery (Department of Health,1993a, p.23). It does not necessarily follow that all 22 per cent would actually choose a home confinement, but it could be assumed that there will be some increase in demand for this service. According to Murphy-Black (1993) it has been suggested that the demand may be in the region of eight per cent of births. As a result of their debate on the Challenges for Nursing and Midwifery (1993) Chief Nursing Officers of England, Wales, Scotland and Northern Ireland assumed that by the year 2001, 15 per cent of births will take place outside hospitals. There is no way of assessing the future demand for home deliveries, but it seems that they will increase and midwifery services will have to be capable of meeting the demand.

To cater for an eight per cent home delivery rate Murphy-Black (1993) predicts that an increased number of midwives would be required, but that this increase could be met by the cost savings which result from the reduced hospital service. She does, however, warn that the absence of any methods of estimating the midwifery hours required to offer the service makes it difficult to argue for such an increase. Caroline Flint (1993) estimates that each woman requires on average 40 hours of midwifery time for her total care from the first antenatal visit to the last postnatal visit. She calculates that a unit with 4,000 deliveries per year would require 139 midwives – 111 with caseloads of approximately 36 women each and 28 midwives as skeleton staff on the labour ward and postnatal ward. These calculations may appear somewhat simple, but Ball et al (1992) gives details of midwives required to provide a comprehensive service within the hospital and community.

There is a possibility of midwives having to deal with unforeseen situations away from the hospital where help and equipment are, in the main, easily accessible. Midwives need to be sufficiently confident to deal effectively and efficiently with any emergency which may arise and have the equipment readily available to allow them to undertake emergency treatment. The obvious skills of resuscitation and management of haemorrhage need to be constantly updated and competence reviewed. Dealing with emergencies in the home will be a situation of which many midwives have little or no experience. Preparation for such a situation needs to be considered.

The provision of back-up services is essential, whether this is the renewal of the obstetric flying squad system or the provision of a paramedic service which is trained to deal with obstetric and neonatal emergencies. The main criticism of such a service is the time taken for them to arrive, and this may be crucial. It is doubtful that paramedic services could manage the situation any better than the adequately trained midwife, but they could offer the essential support and equipment required in many emergency situations and during transfer to hospital.

The debate surrounding home births appears to centre around the issue of safety. The Expert Group addressed this concern and highlighted that safety is often used as a justification for care which women thought unnecessary or distressful. They state, 'Safety is not an absolute concept. It is part of a greater picture encompassing all aspects of health and wellbeing' (p.10). Regarding the risk of home confinement for women with uncomplicated pregnancies, professionals are reminded that the debate on risk has raged for decades with no consensus on the level of risk, and that, '**The inability to reach agreement after this length of time suggests that there is no clear answer**' (p 23).

As previously discussed (Chapter 3) there are no reliable methods of predicting those women who will develop complications other than where abnormalities are present at the start of pregnancy or become apparent during pregnancy. It may be more pertinent to look for ways of identifying those women who will require less intensive monitoring and intervention and allow them the option of choosing where to have their babies. This choice does not have to be made at the beginning of pregnancy. The example of the Isle of Sheppey could be followed. Within this district women, who have previously discussed the options, can make a final decision at any time up to the start of labour whether to have a home birth or a domino delivery (Department of Health, 1993a. p.24). This seems such a simple way of offering a service to women, it removes the pressure on women to make choices early in pregnancy when this may not be the appropriate time and allows time for discussion between the professionals and the woman so that a truly informed decision can be made. It may be that this service could be offered by more midwives throughout the country.

Midwifery-led beds

If, as envisaged, midwives take the role of lead professional for 30 per cent of women, it makes sense that midwives have access to beds within the unit to allow for care of those women who wish to have their babies in hospital. Access to beds by midwives was seen by the Expert Group as a way of preventing women having to visit the hospital in order to reserve a place for delivery. In a hospital oriented service this process makes obvious sense, but as the required shift towards a more community-oriented service (Department of Health, 1993a) takes place, and if women are encouraged to opt for place of delivery any time up to labour commencing, then it is more appropriate that midwives have the use of facilities without resorting to the current system of booking a place in advance. The Report acknowledges that this system is successfully operated at the Royal Berkshire and Battle Hospital NHS Trust, so there is no reason to suppose that it can not operate in other areas.

The advantages of having all the medical services near, should they be required, are apparent, but the hospital environment can remain unwelcoming and frightening to some women who fear loss of control as they enter unfamiliar surroundings. Attempts have been made in many labour wards to create a more homely atmosphere, by installing family rooms, birthing rooms and birthing pools. No doubt many women appreciate these efforts, but having such facilities does not guarantee that care is midwifery led or that women have choice in or control of their care. It is the philosophy of care which needs to be addressed with midwives working with the belief that childbearing is, for the majority of women, a normal physiological process which requires midwifery support and care and not an acute medical condition requiring intensive monitoring and intervention. An alternative to acute unit midwifery led beds is the establishment of midwifery-managed units away from the district general hospital. In the past, these units were defined as General Practitioner Units. Many closed as care became centralized within larger district general hospitals, while some were used solely to provide antenatal care within the local community. As health care is set to become more community-based it may be that these units will in the future provide facilities for intranatal care managed by midwives. Dimond (1994) highlights the concerns of midwives regarding midwifery-managed units, these include risks to mother and baby, transfers from the unit to the district general hospital and litigation. She reassures that many of the fears regarding the safety of the woman and baby are probably felt by midwives in the district general hospitals, and many of the risks are foreseeable with good antenatal screening. If there is no antenatal evidence of risk and some unforeseen event occurs, any civil action is likely to be unsuccessful, provided all reasonable care has been taken. The ability of midwives to deal with emergencies such as resuscitation or haemorrhage and to affect transfer to a district general hospital are areas for which management protocols are required. Professional competence is discussed in Chapter 6.

The arguments regarding the safety of such units have been discredited, (Tew, 1990) but as the Winterton Report (House of Commons, 1992) points out the options for choice by women have been reduced by the closure of these units. With the emphasis of 'Changing Childbirth' (Department of Health, 1993a) on women's choice and control it seems appropriate that they have options other than home or acute hospital delivery.

Choice, control and continuity

Continuity of care requires a philosophical shift on the part of the professionals, starting with the belief that women have the right to make choices and are entitled to influence the care they receive. Continuity of carer demands an appraisal of the ways in which the professionals organize the service. Whatever changes are implemented they should be for the benefit of women.

The whole ethos of 'Changing Childbirth' (Department of Health, 1993a) is that women must have choice in the type of care they receive and have control over the process. In order to have choice women must have alternatives from which to choose and information regarding the benefits and risks to them and their babies of the various options, but most of all they must feel that whatever their choice midwives will support them throughout the childbearing experience. By ensuring that women are encouraged to make informed choices in a supportive and cooperative context they will truly be in control.

CHAPTER SIX

Implications for Practice and Supervision

> From the evidence we received, we recognized that women have great confidence in the midwifery profession. The midwife is able to offer a woman and her family support and encouragement during a time of great change as well as having the clinical skills necessary to determine whether all is progressing normally. Importantly, the midwife is able to work across a variety of settings, and is able to be with the woman when and where needed, ensuring that she remains the focus of care. (Department of Health, 1993a Section 2.11.1 p. 38)

Successive Acts of Parliament have made provision for regulating the practice of midwifery and supervision of midwives, the latest being the Nurses, Midwives and Health Visitors Acts of 1979 and 1992. Under these Acts, provision is made to enable the United Kingdom Central Council (UKCC) to formulate rules regulating the practice of midwives. These rules may in particular;

Section 15. (1)

a)   determine the circumstances by means of which, midwives may be suspended from practice;

b)   require midwives to give notice of their intention to practice to the local supervising authority for the area in which they intend to practice; and

c)   require registered midwives to attend courses of instruction in accordance with the rules.

Nurses, Midwives and Health Visitors Act 1979, Section 15. (1) p.11. In addition to the provision of rules under section 15, there is

provision for general supervision of midwives in section 16.2;
Each local supervising authority shall -

a)   exercise general supervision, in accordance with rules under
     section 15, over all midwives practising within its area;

b)   report any prima facie case of misconduct on the part of a
     midwife which arises in its area to the National Board for the
     part of the United Kingdom in which the authority acts;

c)   have power in accordance with the Council's rules to suspend
     a midwife from practice.

As a result of changes in the structure of the NHS and in the National
Boards, further amendments were made to the 1979 Act in the 1992
Nurses, Midwives and Health Visitors Act. One of these was to
ensure that the function of the National Board in the 1979 Act Section
16-2b is now taken over by the UKCC. There is also a new clause
added to Section 16 of the 1979 Act which states that:

> 16.5) The Council may by rules prescribe standards to be
> observed with respect to advice and guidance provided under
> subsection (4)   (Nurses, Midwives and Health Visitors Act
> 1992, Section 11, p. 6)

Originally in the 1979 Act section 16-4 stated that the National Boards
were responsible for providing the authorities with advice and
guidance but it did not go as far as giving them responsibility for
standard setting. The amendments to the Act have been incorporated
into the Midwives Rules November 1993.

The principal duty of the midwife and the midwifery profession as
a whole is the welfare of the mother and the baby. This being so,
safety is of prime concern but as has been pointed out in the
'Changing Childbirth' report (Department of Health, 1993a, p.10)
'safety is not an absolute concept'. The midwife and the supervisor
of midwives are thus left with a dilemma, particularly when faced
with innovations in practice. The midwife must be able to give the
woman unbiased information and choice in childbirth. This may
lead her to feel uncomfortable or even apprehensive about the
woman's choices. The simple (but mostly inappropriate) solution

would be to take refuge in the tried and tested i.e. the status quo. Until the acceptance of the 'Changing Childbirth' report this might have been fine from the midwife's point of view regardless of the opinion of the woman. Things are not the same now, because if the woman's choice must be respected then the midwife will have to rethink her position and this is where she may need to turn to her supervisor for support. (the report is also Government policy, so Trusts and Purchasers also need to act).

The supervisor of midwives not only has a responsibility to the Local Supervising Authority (LSA) to carry out the statutory functions as laid down in the Nurses, Midwives and Health Visitors Acts (see previous pages). She also has a responsibility to the individual midwives that she supervises under the Code of Practice (UKCC, 1994 , Section 51 p.19) to be a colleague, counsellor and advisor. By so doing she can facilitate changes and innovations in practice. This being so the supervisor can use the legal powers conferred by the Acts to authenticate practice and make it safe for both midwife and woman rather than limiting its scope.

One of the functions of the supervisor of midwives is to maintain standards of midwifery care but before one can maintain a standard one has to identify it and this is where effective supervision is helpful. Supervision of midwives can be an enabling process that assists the individual to consider an innovation in depth, helps set a standard for it, facilitates its implementation and evaluates its effectiveness. This is extremely important where the proposal is at the cutting edge of practice because under Rule 40 (2),

> A practising midwife must not, except in an emergency, undertake any treatment which she has not been trained to give either before or after registration as a midwife and which is outside her sphere of practice. (UKCC Midwives Rules, 1993, p.20)

Under this rule no procedure or innovation is possible unless it has already been implemented, tried and tested elsewhere. Generally speaking most practices that midwives will want to undertake will fall into this category. However, there may be some that will not. Water birth in its early days fell into this category for most midwives.

The supervisor can enable practice by assisting the midwife to research the subject thoroughly, give the benefit of advice, enlist the support of the appropriate services and, if necessary, be physically present at the innovation and last but not least can act as an advocate for both the midwife and the mother.

It is interesting to note that the UKCC. have fully supported midwives in the recognition that water birth is 'an alternative method of care and one which must therefore fall within the normal sphere of the practice of a midwife'. (UKCC 16/1994). Council suggests that the midwife discusses the matter with her supervisor of midwives in order to seek further professional advice and makes a record of the discussion. Being mindful of the right to choose the Council states that it is the duty of the supervisor of midwives to ensure that local policies are formulated with the advice of practising midwives and supervisors of midwives and that such policies ensure the midwife has support in all settings. It concludes that employing authorities will wish to develop local policies and that the Council considers it essential that supervisors of midwives and practising midwives are actively involved in their development.

The ten criteria for success outlined in the 'Changing Childbirth' report (Dept of Health, 1993a, p. 70) in themselves constitute measurable standards of care for the maternity services, but just how they will be achieved will be left to the midwives within the service to decide for themselves. The indicators of success do not in themselves detail the standards of the service to be provided but in the action for change 5.2.4 it states;

> Both purchasers and providers should provide clear information for users about the services available to them, and the standards they should expect. They should take a much more critical approach to the effectiveness of different practices and techniques (Department of Health, 1993a, p. 69).

Leading the work on setting of standards will be the responsibility of the supervisor of midwives. This will involve a thorough understanding of the issues involved and a reappraisal of midwifery guidelines, policies and procedures. These will need to be reviewed and evaluated for adequacy and suitability in the light of the recommendations of the report. Standards are usually based on outcomes of midwifery care and so these can be devised in conjunction with the users of the service e.g. local groups or in close collaboration with the maternity service liaison committee, based on the targets for achievemnet for developing woman centred care. The Donabedian model (1969) is often used in the NHS and has the advantage of being outcome driven but caution is necessary in that it is essential that the outcomes are specific to the philosophy of 'Changing Childbirth' and are woman focused. The standards should also be cognisant of current research. All midwives should be involved in the devising of the standards in a bottom up approach that will be far more effective than a top down imposition. They should also be involved in the audit of the standards and implement subsequent changes.

Standard setting is only one aspect of the role of the supervisor of midwives. Another major area is that of facilitating practice and being a support for the midwife. One of the duties that is undertaken on behalf of the LSA is ensuring that midwives have notified their intention to practice. Another is that of interviewing midwives with regard to their learning needs. The supervisor and the midwife should ideally have a meeting at least once a year when practice issues are discussed. The supervisor must assure herself that the midwife is in a position to notify her intention to practice i.e. she is actually functioning as a midwife. This is not as trite a statement as it first appears because there are midwives working as practice nurses or educationalists who have to safeguard their right to notify their intention to practice very carefully. The Midwives Rules state quite categorically that a practising midwife:

> means a midwife who attends professionally upon a woman during the antenatal, intranatal and/or postnatal period or who holds a post for which a midwifery qualification is essential and who notifies her intention to practice to the local supervising authority (UKCC, November 1993 p.8).

This rule not only ensures that the midwife maintains her skills and right to practice but also protects the public in that no professional can act as a midwife unless they fulfil the criteria to be a practising midwife and they have a supervisor of midwives.

The 'Changing Childbirth' report highlighted several areas where it is felt there is a need for more in service education e.g.

communication skills (Department of Health,1993a, p.57). It is the role of the supervisor to identify these needs in greater depth and to enable the midwife to take advantage of existing training opportunities. Where there is an identified need and no programme in existence, the supervisor should work with the midwifery managers and the Approved Teacher of the educational establishment to plan appropriate study days and skills workshops for the staff. The supervisor can also work with the Trust training department to plan in house developments.

Not only must the supervisor work with midwives on an individual basis she must also have a watching eye on the service as a whole. She must scan the existing provision with regard to existing facilities and the changes that will be required with the implementation of the 'Changing Childbirth report and ensure that there is no shortfall in the interim period. For example, in many areas there is an obstetric flying squad in existence. It has been highlighted that these will soon be obsolete. However, where they exist they must be kept in operation until there is a fully functioning paramedic service to take its place. Otherwise a midwife may find herself in the position of having to deal with an obstetric emergency without a backup service. If the supervisor allows this to happen not only will she be party to the compromising of safety standards for the individual mother and baby, she will also have let the midwife down and will have failed to fulfil her statutory obligation under the Nurses, Midwives and Health Visitors Acts. She must also ensure that in changing times no other person takes on the role of a practising midwife.

The supervisors in each district will therefore have to make absolutely sure that there are protocols in place to deal with the obstetric emergencies that may arise. As 'Changing Childbirth' becomes more and more of a reality, there is bound to be an increase in community based care and so there will be more chance of problems arising in the community. Haemorrhage, shock and neonatal asphyxia are the first that spring to mind and it is a practice/ supervision issue to ensure that all professional groups are provided with guidelines for action. This will include ensuring that midwives as well as paramedics can set up intravenous infusions and are up to date in both maternal and neonatal resuscitation. The setting up of an intravenous infusion in the community by the midwife is being debated at the moment. Some supervisors are against it on the grounds that the midwife in the community should have the backing of a readily accessible paramedic service at all times and so should never be in the position of needing to do this herself. Others would not agree and would see it as an essential skill. The important point is that, whatever decision is made, the safety of the mother must not be in jeopardy and there must be locally agreed standards that ensure that an IV infusion if needed can be sited within minutes.

Most supervisors would be very wary of all paramedics having a week long obstetric training as happens in some areas. The argument against this is that paramedics should only be delivering a baby in an emergency and should not be undertaking any other duties that need obstetric training. These are within the role of the midwife or doctor. Paramedics will need to be educated or updated in emergency delivery techniques and will need specific guidelines regarding their role in particular emergencies. One such emergency that will constitute a practice/supervision issue is the case of the woman with severe pregnancy induced hypertension or one who is having an eclamptic fit. Paramedics are not trained to distinguish this from a epileptic grand mal seizure and it will be up to the supervisors of midwives in conjunction with the obstetricians to draw up a protocol for action in such a case. Previously the obstetric flying squad came out to the woman and she was not moved until she had been heavily sedated by an obstetrician. It is likely that the protocol will ensure that it is the midwife who sedates the woman, perhaps using rectal diazepam or something similar. The supervisor must also ensure that any policies that are agreed for the paramedical service in relation to childbirth are supportive of the midwife. For example, it must be the midwife's decision to admit the woman to hospital and if she considers this a necessity the paramedics must not be able to argue against or override her decision. Another supportive function of the paramedic service is that of carrying necessary drugs. In some areas it is extremely dangerous on a personal level for midwives to carry drugs, particularly controlled drugs. They are at risk of physical violence and damage to their cars in order to make them hand over drugs and needles (Gill, 1994).

In most areas the paediatric flying squad will no longer be functional. It is the responsibility of the supervisors of midwives to ensure that the midwife has the backing of the paramedics and that every midwife has the skill necessary to maintain the child's condition until it is transferred to hospital by the paramedics. She must also ensure that there is a unit policy or system in place that ensures the midwife is able and knows how to directly contact the appropriate neonatal services. Good communication in this instance is vital.

Both the 'Changing Childbirth ' report (Department of Health, 1993a) and the 'Winterton' report (House of Commons, 1991–2) advocate the continuance of midwife/general practitioner led units as part of the woman's menu of choice. The 'Changing Childbirth' report is quoted as saying that there is;

> no clear statistical evidence that having their babies away from general hospital maternity units is less safe for women with uncomplicated pregnancies (Department of Health, 1993a, 'Changing Childbirth' section 2.6.6. p.23).

However, there is still a voice of caution needed for as the latest information on NHS risk management (NHS Management Executive, 1993) points out managers should satisfy themselves that there are adequate arrangements for cover by medical and other staff. This is not only a managerial issue but a supervision one also because if the cover is not available the midwife may find herself working in unsafe practice conditions.

Obstetric emergencies are just part of the overall practice matters that will need to be addressed in the implementation of the 'Changing Childbirth' report. Supervisors of midwives will be in the forefront of identifying from a practice position just how the service can be woman focused. This will involve using their local knowledge of particular groups and facilitating the identification of the special needs of such groups. The supervisors will help the midwives as they develop their teams and be involved in establishing good practice. For example, one area of good practice is the establishment of pre pregnancy clinics based in the community. According to Lindsay Smith (Chamberlain and Patel, 1994 p.112) there are no randomized controlled trials on the effectiveness of pre pregnancy clinics to improve fetal outcome. However many professionals would see the establishment of a clinic or drop in centre that gives advice prior to pregnancy on the dangers of smoking, alcohol, rubella etc. as eminently sensible. Indeed the Department of Health has recently (July, 1994) announced a grant of £15,000 to Solihull maternity hospital in order that it can develop such a service. Another aspect is the determination of criteria, as part of a multidisciplinary collaboration, for identifying women suitable for midwifery practice development units.

As the midwifery teams develop and organize their caseloads and care practices in the community, there are some specific issues that will need the skills of the supervisor. The establishment of teams inevitably necessitate a different pattern of working in order that continuity of care and carer can be achieved. Midwives will be called upon to be more flexible and established shift patterns will no longer suffice. Many midwives are concerned about the effect of such working patterns upon their private life and even upon their ability to continue to work as a midwife and of course clinical grading and the pay scale is of paramount concern. However, it is the responsibility of the supervisor to ensure two things in relation to this. Firstly that every pregnant, labouring and postnatal woman can always be assured of the services of a midwife as and when required. The other issue for the supervisor is that the team is large enough and organized enough to be able to give cover to the number of women that it has booked. There is also a recommendation for good practice that two midwives attend a home confinement. This would mean that sickness, holiday, student mentorship requirements and staff development needs are accounted for in the final numbers. It is a practice/supervision issue in that the supervisor must be certain that midwives will never be so flexible that they are working such long hours that safe care is jeopardised. However, the undetermined factor at this moment is; How long can a midwife work and still be considered safe and whose decision is it to determine this? The preceding comments apply to all midwifery teams but one important consideration is that of the independent midwife. It may be that the midwife works in a very small team or is a completely independent agent and the supervisor will have to satisfy herself that the continuity of care and carer is a safe option.

The supervisor of midwives must also ensure that not only is practice safe for the mother and the baby but that it is safe for the midwife as well. This includes the actual physical safety of the midwife. The days seem to be long gone when a midwife in uniform was free to go into the roughest area alone at night. There have been reports of midwives being stabbed or dragged from their cars whilst on duty in the community (Gill, 1994). As the implementation of 'Changing Childbirth' will inevitably mean that more midwives are working in the community and also that they are bound by the Midwives Rules (1993, Rule 40) to provide care their safety has to be a supervision issue. (Obviously it is mainly an employment and managerial issue under the Health and Safety at Work Act (Department of Employment, 1974)). Gill (1994) recommends that several measures are introduced including better communication so that the midwife will know that she is actually going out to a genuine case, better liaison with the police, provision of two way radios and personal alarms, and visiting in pairs particularly in vulnerable areas. It behoves the supervisors of each locality to ensure that there is a good communication network and safety protocols in place in order that the midwife is as safe as possible and that no avoidable incidents take place.

A supervision/practice issue to be considered in the development of 'Changing Childbirth' is the proficiency of the midwife. Although midwives working within most hospital settings tend to rotate around the clinical areas and so develop and maintain their proficiency in the all round care of the childbearing woman, this is not true of all midwives. Some midwives have tended to work mainly in one area of practice and so may be less than proficient in some areas of care. This may include hospital midwives who have not worked in the community since they were students, or visa versa, community midwives who have not worked in the hospital setting for many a year. The supervisors along with the managers will consider the competencies that are absolutely necessary for the 'generic' midwife and ensure that midwives are proficient in the necessary skills before working in the community and undertaking home confinements. This will probably extend to midwives working in midwifery practice development units. The midwife may need an updating programme which gives her, for example, time on the labour ward reacquainting herself with delivery techniques and/or perineal suturing techniques. However accountability for her practice remains with the midwife. The supervisor cannot assume vicarious liability for the midwife's actions.

The midwife must also be aware of the role and function of the supervisor of midwives and know how to contact her as necessary. (It may mean that there is a rota of supervisors on call). The supervisor must ensure that the midwife's record keeping is impeccable and that her bags are correctly and well stocked with in date drugs and up to date equipment. Likewise the midwife needs to know how to obtain stocks and drugs. In the case of independent midwives, the supervisor must satisfy herself that the midwife has a suitable means of sterilization of equipment and disposal of the placenta. If she does not, the supervisor will usually facilitate an arrangement between the midwife and the appropriate hospital departments. She must also satisfy herself that the midwife has the support of a general practitioner and knows how to transfer the woman's care if a complication arises.

As the number of home confinements increase, there is a statistical probability that at sometime either sooner or later a baby will be born stillborn. The woman and her family will need a great deal of physical and emotional support from the midwife at such a time. She will have to lay the baby out and help the parents, siblings and grandparents in the grieving process. This is emotionally draining for the midwife at any time but if it is an unexpected stillbirth, she will also have emotions that are particular to herself. For example, she may blame herself either rightly or wrongly and will be in need of personal support at this time. She must be able to turn to her supervisor for this and for the knowledge which will help her come to terms with the event and her part in it. If there is any doubt about the safety of the midwife's practice she may become the centre of an inquiry which could possibly lead to disciplinary action or suspension from practice. The supervisor will act as a colleagues, counsellor and advisor in this case even though another supervisor of midwives may be involved in the investigation aspect.

The supervisor of midwives has a duty to ensure that all practice is safe and this is particularly important where midwives are working in independant ways outside the health service. It may be that a supervisor has to deal with a perceived lack of good practice for example as a result of a general practitioner's (or a member of the public) complaint. It is usually the role of the manager in the first instance but in the case of an independent midwife, it will be solely the supervisor. If there is any justification in the complaint,the midwife may be reported to the Local Supervising Authority (LSA) and put on supervised practice whereby her theoretical and clinical competence to practice is assessed or she may even be suspended from practice by the LSA whilst an investigation is pending. A supervisor of midwives will act on behalf of the LSA.as an investigating officer but another supervisor will act as a support for the midwife at this time.

The supervisor of midwives should work with other members of the multidisciplinary team in the monitoring and auditing of the standards of practice and the woman's satisfaction with the service. Earlier it was stated that an important feature of supervision was the facilitation of the setting of standards for good practice. This being so the audit of the practice will enable the individual midwives to gain a three dimensional view of the service they provide. It will also enable women to feed back into the system and make their needs felt. Audit of practice from the supervision angle will ensure that women are given individualized care which is research based, effective and can be an agent for change. In this way the practice will be truly woman centred and in a cyclical fashion, can be used to further set standards which will ensure that women's needs are not only assessed but acted upon and as far as possible met.

The role of the obstetric Senior House officer (SHO) has been considered by the Expert Group to be necessary of re-examination. Two points that will involve the supervisor of midwives is the suggestion that experienced midwives may become more formally involved in their training. The educational aspect will be more fully covered in a later chapter. However, for the supervisor it will may mean that more support is given to the midwife in this role. A system of teaching and assessment of the doctor will need to be formulated and responsibility and accountability determined. This will be particularly necessary when both the midwife and the obstetric senior house officer attend a woman in childbirth. It is highly likely that the midwife will be the lead and named professional and the obstetric SHO will act in the role of student. However, a clearly defined policy and protocol must be developed before a problem arises.

There are issues surrounding care in the community which the supervisor of midwives must satisfy herself that women will receive the best possible care. At first some of these may seem to be outside the remit of the supervisor but on further examination they prove not to be. One of these is the issue of the cessation of the obstetric flying squad. Midwives will have to carry more equipment. This has a cost implication but it will be part of the policy making role of the supervisor to determine the minimum requirements. It may be that general practitioners will employ their own midwife and if so the supervisor will need to ensure that the midwife is eligible and competent to practice. Other issues include the clarification of the role of the midwife as the lead professional or named midwife. At this moment there are conflicting views from various parts of the country. It is likely that protocols need drawing up with regard to transfer of care from one professional to another.

Monitoring and audit of practice and practice areas are a supervision/ practice matter and the supervisor will ensure at regular intervals that the conditions and practice are conducive to safe care. Overall as there is such a heavy responsibility for safe practice borne by supervisors of midwives, it is necessary that they themselves have a supportive mechanism. They need to be selected very carefully and this is under debate at the moment by the midwifery profession and by the UKCC. Also under discussion is the thorny question of their assessment of competence in the role, and their deselection if necessary. There is lack of consistency and uniformity of the practice of supervision across the United Kingdom and this will need to be resolved. Another matter that has never been a problem until now is the matter of funding for supervision. As this is a statutory function, there is a case for separate funding which would ensure that all members of the midwifery profession, whoever their employer may be, will not be disadvantaged regarding their freedom to undertake the role.

CHAPTER SEVEN

Purchasing and Contracting Issues

Purchasers should:

> develop strategic plans for maternity services, with guidance
> on future purchasing intentions showing positive moves
> towards women-centred and community-based care.
> (Department of Health, 1993a, 'Changing Childbirth' Chapter
> 4, p. 60)

In the past ten years there has not only been a reformation in the
delivery of maternity services but also a huge change in the structure
of the National Health Service as a whole. The move towards the
internal market began with the reforms outlined in the Government
white paper 'Working for Patients' (Department of Health, 1989).
This was followed by Working Paper 1 'Self Governing hospitals'
(NHS, 1989) which proposed the institution of hospitals as self-
governing and separate legal organizations within the NHS. It was
made law in the NHS and Community Care Act of 1990 which
enshrined the principle of competition as the motivating factor in
the assurance of quality care. A large number of hospitals are now
hospital Trusts but some discrete services such as the community
services have also been granted Trust status.

The Trusts are self-managed by a board of directors chaired by a
person appointed and accountable to the secretary of state for health.
The Trust boards have far more autonomy than hospital management
boards or Health Authorities prior to the reforms. These powers
include amongst others the right to determine their own staffing
ratios and the staff's terms and conditions of service, the right to
dispose of property as they see fit, determine contracts for services
and to generate income. However they are still fully within the NHS
and are still governed by much of the law affecting the NHS. The

creation of Trusts is aimed at improving the quality, efficiency and cost-effectiveness of the service provided, so an internal market culture has come into existence, with the Trusts assuming the role of healthcare providers. The Trusts operate in a competitive climate and by acting as businesses they can respond to local needs and be both effective and efficient. If they do not, they, like any other inefficient business, may not survive. This being so, one of their main objectives is to provide a quality service and the maternity service is no exception. Independent midwives could also act as providers except that they are not considered to be 'Health Service Bodies' under the National Health Service and Community Care Act 1990 but some are in group practices that are negotiating on a sub-contractual basis. One example is the South East London Midwifery Group Practice which has been granted initial Regional funding. Independent midwives give holistic/continuity of care and would be well placed to act as providers and give more choice to women but it is unlikely in the short term because it will need a change in the law to enable them to contract directly with the purchaser (Warren, 1994).

The other half of the business partnership is the purchaser. These are the general practitioner fund-holders and the purchasing authorities who may be the District Health Authority or a consortium. At the moment fund-holding general practitioners do not buy maternity services. However it is possible in the future that parts of the service could be contracted out. Experimental work is being undertaken as part of locality purchasing pilot projects where GPs determine which services will be provided by whom, and at what cost on behalf of the purchasers – maternity services being one such service. The government have already said that they 'wish to see GP fund-holders exerting greater power in the internal market' (Tyler and Jenkins, 1994). There is concern about this and the Royal College of Midwives will only support it if fundholding is restricted to GPs purchasing continuous packages of maternity care from a range of providers. For the time being at least the purchasing consortiums are continuing to buy the maternity services as an integrated package. The main aim of the purchaser is to ensure that the money available will be spent to the best advantage. This being so the services available are evaluated, expert clinical advice is sought and the contract will be given to the provider who is both cost-effective and ensures high quality health care delivery.

There are two parts to purchasing, which are commissioning and contracting. The purchaser commissions the service which in the case of the maternity service will be based upon the ideals of 'Changing Childbirth' and enters into a contract with the provider unit for the supply of a high-class service catering for the needs of local women. The purchaser is in command of the budget for buying maternity services and so is in control and will be instrumental in assuring that the Health Service reforms are implemented. These include the Health of the Nation (Department of Health, 1992a) key strategies, the implementation of the Patient's Charter (Department of Health, 1991) and the Patient's Charter: the Maternity Services (Department of Health, 1994), and of course the action points and indicators of success in 'Changing Childbirth'.

Although the details of the contracting process will vary from place to place there is a general pattern that is common to all. The first part of the process is the development by the purchaser of a strategic framework. This will form the basis of the contract and details the service and standards that will be required. The purchaser will usually liaise with local consumers and the Maternity Service Liaison Committee (MSLC) in order to develop the blueprint. Some of the ways that this is achieved is through 'local voice initiatives', 'focus groups', consumer surveys and clinical audit.

'Local voice initiatives' is one way of describing efforts by bodies such as the Regional Health Authority to determine the views of service users. Very often in the past the views of local women were either not sufficiently documented or were acquired in a patchy unrepresentative and unsolicitated manner. In order to overcome such problems some authorities have made monies available for reliable and valid research into women's perceptions of the maternity service.

One such project is project 'Liverbirth' which has been commissioned by the Liverpool Health Authorities. It involves two research projects, one a qualitative and the other a quantitative study which focuses on the 'wishes and views of the women of Liverpool on a neighbourhood basis' (Guelbert, 1994). This project is concerned with the views of women on pregnancy, the choice of carer, site of care, records, parentcraft, information and explanation, labour/childbirth – place of delivery and the postnatal period. It makes recommendations in 'the context of a philosophy consistent with the spirit of "Cumberlege" within the framework of neighbourhood planning; and with a view to achieving the long-term aim of "Project Liverbirth"'(Guelbert, 1994).

The Winterton report recommended that the government strengthen the role of the Maternity Services Liaison Committees (MSLCs) because they have the potential at local level to 'channel more effectively user's views into the planning and monitoring stages of service delivery' (1992, para 445). This strengthening is under way in most parts of the country and the MSLCs are becoming more effective.

The National Childbirth Trust (NCT) (which is one of the most influential maternity services consumer organizations in the country) in conjunction with the Greater London Association of Community Health Councils has recently published a briefing paper entitled the `Maternity Service Liaison Committees – A forum for Change (Lewison, 1994). This is concerned that 'There is scant evidence about the effectiveness of MSLCs' (p. 3) and quotes Jo Garcia (1987) who says 'There is no systematic evidence about the ways that MSLC.s work. Anecdotal evidence suggests that some are very successful while others are troubled by tensions between interest groups or individuals, or lack of any clear direction'. This report is concerned about the ambivalent status of the MSLC as is highlighted in the Royal College of Midwives guidelines (RCM, 1993) which sees them as sitting somewhere in the middle and acting as a channel of communication for purchasers, providers and users of the maternity services. Instead (according to this report) the MSLC should be firmly sited with the District Health Authority as purchasers in order to be completely effective.

As the purchaser needs to involve users of the service, the MSLC can enable this process if it itself is properly representative of the community. It can be so by involving members from local voluntary organizations, the Community Health Council, individual users of the service and consumer organizations such as the National Childbirth Trust as well as members from the professional groups. In this way women can be involved from the very beginning and the following objective can be achieved:

> Users of maternity services should be actively involved in planning and reviewing services. The lay representation must reflect the ethnic, cultural and social mix of the local population. A maternity services liaison committee should be established within every district health authority. ('Changing Childbirth', section 3.2, p. 47)

One of the issues for the 'Changing Childbirth' report and for the establishment of an effective MSLC is the inclusion of representatives from the ethnic minority groups within the community. It is imperative that ways are sought to involve people who do not normally take part in formal consumer groups. Some areas have developed focus groups which concentrate on particular sections of the community and by using questionnaires or in depth interviews can assess the needs of particular sections of the community.

As previously stated the effective MSLC will also involve members of the various professional groups including midwifery managers, supervisors of midwives, midwife educationalists, obstetricians, paediatrician and general practitioners, members of the Family Health Services Authority, the purchasing authority, Trust Board representatives and the social services. It will provide the platform for discussion and will review information available for mothers and current practice. It will also explore ways of ensuring that local people can give their views on the maternity services and will monitor services against the indicators of success in the 'Changing Childbirth' report. By being firmly allied to the health Authority the MSLC can be very effective in the management of change because it will be instrumental in the development of the strategic framework for purchasing.

The strategic framework is in some ways a blueprint for the contract. The purchasing authority will be working from principles based on the philosophy of the 'Changing Childbirth' report. These will be seeking to ensure that there is accessibility, community care and sensitivity to local needs, and that the woman is the focus of care, has choice, continuity, control and involvement. There will be a summary of the service to be provided and detailed specifications with regard to users needs, e.g. women should have:

1. Information services on place of birth, options on the place of birth and the lead professional.
2. Opportunities to discuss care plans and time to make or change decisions.
3. Access to a midwife and be able to book with a midwife.
4. The right to carry her own case notes.
5. Full information regarding her care and the right to be involved when decisions are made about her care.
6. The right to individualize care and her wishes included in a birth plan.
7. Appropriate antenatal care.
8. The name of a local midwife, who is known to her and who she can ask for advice.
9. Support and continuity of care in labour.
10. Flexibility of stay in hospital postnatally.
11. The support of the midwife, obstetrician, GP and health visitor as required.
12. Information postnatally on infant care and feeding, contraception and health education.

The purchaser may ask for a report from the provider units on their proposals for delivering the maternity services in the light of 'Changing Childbirth' and require information on antenatal, intranatal and postnatal care, parentcraft and health education, available options for place of birth, innovations in practice and the supporting facilities, e.g. water birth and the presence of a birthing pool, and protocols for obstetric emergencies. They will also need information on staff education and training programmes particularly in relation to counselling, interpersonal skills and programmes designed to help staff understand the needs of and be able to support women whose first language is not English or women who have special needs, e.g. the deaf woman.

The purchaser may also as part of the contract specification build in an assurance that liaison will occur between itself, the provider, the local Community Health Council, the MSLC and consumer groups to ensure that local user's views are constantly sought and taken account of in the process.

Other aspects of the contract specification will include local service elements and activity levels of service. Local service elements will include provisions such as pre- pregnancy advice, screening tests, antenatal monitoring, inductions of labour and care after delivery. Activity levels of service are statistical performance indicators, e.g. number and percentage of hospital, domino or home confinements, midwife and obstetrician cases, number of antenatal attendances and postnatal visits, and so on. The precise population served and the demographic area will be identified as well as a projection of future trends. The volume of women to be catered for by the contract will be calculated by estimating the number who are expected to deliver within and outside the catchment area. One of the key areas in contracts during the next five years will be the achievement of the 'Changing Childbirth' indicators of success (see Appendix I).

The development of the service specification is only part of the contracting process which takes place over a year. The contracting timetable usually starts in September with the production of the strategic framework. Between October and December the senior midwives, obstetricians and business managers of the provider units will meet to examine the strategic framework and consider their ability to provide the services as requested. There may be some negotiation and shift of position on either side at this time. It is important that it is not seen as a process involving opponents but rather as a way that both sides can ensure improvements in the maternity services. During this time there will be discussions on price per maternity episode, volume, payment and quality assurance mechanisms. The provider will supply the purchaser with detailed prices and will 'be related to various activity levels and will cover the cost of providing the services, including staff, equipment, buildings etc,' (Morris-Thompson, 1994).

During January, February and March the financial negotiations between the purchasers and providers are completed and the resources are allocated by the Regional to the District Health Authorities. The contract teams meet to examine the prices in detail and to negotiate the type of contract which according to Coats (Chamberlain and Patel, 1994, pp. 132–34) can be a cost and volume, cost per case or a block contract. The cost and volume contract is one where payment is related to agreed activity levels whereas the cost per case contract is one where the cost of each individual patient is calculated and charged to the purchaser. The block contract is the one most usual for the maternity services and specifies facilities, work load agreements and activity levels of service within agreed specifications. The provider unit receives payment in instalments from the purchaser. The difficulty for the purchaser is that much is taken on good faith as the payment is made regardless of activity and so it is up to the provider to ensure that the contract is honoured. The advantage for the provider is that it is gives flexibility to cope with peaks and troughs in the number and types of maternity episode to be dealt with. A block contract with indicative volumes will usually overcome this issue. The negotiations culminate in the signing of the contracts which is usually completed by 31 March.

The Health Authority has a duty to provide a comprehensive maternity service so in some ways the providers are almost guaranteed a contract, except where there is more than one provider unit locally. However 'Changing Childbirth' is now Government policy and so the provider has to demonstrate how it can achieve the indicators of success. Many of the provider units have formed project teams to plan, develop and implement the requirements of 'Changing Childbirth'. These include developing a way of standardization of record-keeping and the formulation of hand-held case notes. A notable example of this is the work undertaken in Milton Keynes (Fawdrey, 1994) on pregnancy health records which standardizes the case notes carried by a pregnant woman and collects the information in a comprehensive and significantly different manner. There is also work being undertaken to develop a national hand-held maternity record.

The project groups are working hard to develop team midwifery and develop a system whereby each mother can be assured of being able to book with a midwife as the lead professional if she so wishes, and once booked will be have a named midwife who is responsible for her care and who she can turn to for advice. Team midwifery to date has been implemented in many ways and some of the project teams have found the information in Mapping Team Midwifery (Institute of Manpower Studies, 1993) useful. Also by sharing ideas they have stopped themselves from 'reinventing the wheel'. For example, some of the pilot schemes have identified problems such as the difficulty in determining the ideal ratio of midwives to women. Another problem that has been highlighted by a pilot scheme is the danger of allocating too many midwives to the team and leaving the rest of the unit short-staffed. The Christmas and New Year holidays also posed a problem for one unit. Two teams had to amalgamate over the period and this in itself caused some friction. There have also been problems with identifying the right skill mix of midwives, i.e. numbers of E, F or G grades in the team and the exact meaning of carrying a case load or utilizing the midwifery skills within the framework of clinical grading. Clinical grading is a major problem for all concerned because being as it is designed for nurses in a hierarchical setup it mitigates against midwives who can take on the role from the point of registration.

Project work is only one part of the venture on the part of the provider units. The key to the development is in an multidisciplinary approach involving midwives, obstetricians, business managers and the general practitioners. The approach favoured by several units is to set up a steering group to identify the innovation and its aims in relation to the 'Changing Childbirth' report. Planning the innovation involves consultation with all levels of the organization and ideally being driven by the staff themselves. Key areas that need agreement are the role of the midwife, general practitioner and obstetrician and the clarification of the identification, responsibility and transfer of the lead professional. Setting up of midwifery practice units and/or access to midwifery led beds is another area that must have joint agreement and clear guidelines for usage. Policies and protocols will have to be designed and approved to cover the type of woman admitted to the midwifery practice units. Risk assessment and referral procedures will have to be agreed and resources identified and allocated. Clinical practices will be scrutinised to ensure that the care is research-based, appropriate, woman focused and community centred. Methods of determining the named midwife and ensuring objective unbiased information are also issues that need to be considered if the target of enabling 75 per cent of women to know the person who cares for them during their delivery is achieved. This in itself is not as easy as it seems because as yet there are many interpretations of what 'know' means (Jackson, 1994) who also considers that unbiased information is an ideal that we are striving for but for the moment perhaps the best we can probably achieve is a balanced opinion.

Many of the provider units are now at the point of demonstrating to the purchasers their plans for delivering the service. However there are aspects that will be ongoing and present either teething problems that can be resolved or major stumbling blocks that will need a complete rethink. One of the potential problems will be that of finance and resource allocation. If the service is woman focused it may be that women fall into two camps, those that wish high tech care and those that want low intervention one to one care. Fears have already been raised on this issue, Walkinshaw (Chamberlain and Patel, 1994, p. 130) considers that this issue must be addressed within the new structure. Resources are finite and he poses the question as to whether society would want monitors thrown away or anaesthetists sacked in order to deliver one to one care. This may be far too black and white a dilemma but it is highly likely that there are shades of grey around these problems. One thing is certain and it is that interprofessional rivalries can play no part in determining the resource allocation. To be effective the maternity service must be costed with efficiency and quality care as the goals. It is highly likely that this will mean a maternity service which offers the woman a community-based system of continuity of care and carer with the full back up services of a consultant unit.

Some of the teething problems centre around achieving some of the objectives for providers in 'Changing Childbirth' such as reviewing the pattern of antenatal care and parentcraft education sessions. It may be quite difficult to persuade women that they do not need to be seen as often in pregnancy as they have up to now. This may be so because women want more from the visit than just a physical checkup. Methven (1989) found that little attention was paid to women's psychosocial situation and perhaps this needs to be addressed with the role of the midwife and the purpose of antenatal care revisited by research. Booking visits are conducted in the women's home in some places and it may be that there is a case for more antenatal care being given in the home. Also there may be a few operational problems, e.g. changing the times of parentcraft sessions and persuading midwives to deliver different content in a more user friendly manner. Midwives may be rather reluctant to conduct deliveries at home and will need support and inservice education in order to feel confident and to achieve competency.

One objective in 'Changing Childbirth' for providers is that they should establish mechanisms for identifying women with more complex needs than are normally encountered' (Chapter 3 p. 46). These needs may vary and may include women with physical problems, e.g. wheelchair bound, young teenage mothers, those who cannot speak English, travellers, those with learning difficulties and people who are socially disadvantaged. Schemes to identify and access these women are varied. In some parts of the country midwives are holding awareness sessions in high street stores and attending community centres and shopping malls, e.g. the William Smellie Maternity Unit roadshow. Some areas have aquanatal sessions run by midwives where they can meet and hold meetings with local women. Some, like the UCL hospitals, have drawn up detailed equal access policy and codes of practice and/or have advocacy workers. This aims to ensure that 'factors such as race, colour, religion, nationality, ethnicity and ability in English, homelessness and disability do not affect the quality of service received' (UCL, 1994). It is concerned with such factors as the problems that non-English-speaking women have with discussing maternity care, discrimination and the Race Relations Act 1976 and also with practical issues such as the problems of getting an adequate diet when one is homeless or the fear of not being seen as a fit parent if one is disabled.

Other objectives in the Report will be less difficult for the providers to achieve. These include:

- Having agreed guidelines for the care of women in labour which include guidance on obtaining anaesthetic and paediatric advice.
- Monitoring patterns of feeding and assessing whether women are receiving the appropriate advice and feel confident with the method chosen.
- Ensuring that advice from a paediatrician is available as required to a midwife working in the community.
- Ensuring that there are appropriate up dating programmes for midwives who are moving into new areas of practice.

Most of these kind of recommendations will be achieved by the provider unit senior personnel meeting together and drawing up workable protocols and guidelines and ensuring that there is good communication to all the practitioners involved. However some will only be achieved through detailed service monitoring and evaluation.

Monitoring and evaluation is performed by assessing performance against the agreed standards on a regular basis. It is usual in the provider units to have quality assurance/audit departments which are responsible for much of the work involved but in reality quality is the responsibility of everyone. Monitoring of the contract will be undertaken by the purchasers in an agreed manner, for example, it may be that a quarterly report is required, specifying achievement to date of all the targets including the 'Changing Childbirth' Indicators of success. It may mean monthly visits (or more) to the unit to assess whether there is evidence of compliance with the standards. Patient activity returns will be scrutinised as will reports on service reviews and improvements. Feedback from consumer organisations such as the Community Health Councils will be taken into account as will the review of the maternity services by the MSLC.

Some of the statistical indicators, e.g. number of caesarean sections, home confinements, number of complaints, perinatal and maternal mortality are very straightforward to audit. Most of the indicators of success in 'Changing Childbirth' such as 30 per cent of women being admitted under the care of a midwife can be included in this but the 'soft' indicators are less straightforward. It will mean more than a simple set of statistics to determine whether every knows one midwife who ensures continuity of care.

Similarly there are standards in the Patient's Charter (Department of Health, 1991) and the Patient's Charter and the Maternity Services (Department of Health, 1994) which must be monitored which are less easy to audit. For example, one of the Patient's Charter standards is respect for privacy, dignity and religious and cultural beliefs. One way of auditing this standard is by using a compliance tool as does the Suffolk Health Authority which identifies the purchaser's expectations and looks for evidence of practice and monitors compliance on the day that the purchaser makes its visit. Below 90 per cent is considered non-compliance. Norwich Health Authority uses a different type of audit tool whereby such matters as the height of doors to toilets can be assessed and ticked off on an audit form. Other Authorities use a Donabedian style, structure, process and outcome audit form. Some of the softer outcomes are reliant on consumer satisfaction surveys which are more often than not in questionnaire form (which, of course, will only receive answers to questions that are asked). Providers may be required as part of the contract to undertake a certain number of these surveys per year.

Also part of the evaluation process is that of clinical audit. which is 'the systematic and critical analysis of the quality of care' (Department of Health, 1993d). This is a professional activity and the midwives, obstetricians, paediatricians, radiologists, anaesthetists etc are all involved in scrutinizing maternity care outcomes in order to improve the care given. Since April 1991 each Family Health Service Authority (FHSA) has been required to set up a Medical Audit Advisory Group with the remit of encouraging every practitioner to become involved in audit activity. Funding has been given to the Regional Health Authorities and Royal Colleges to finance the implementation of a systematic method of audit. Systems are being developed to establish a common method of data collection and communication between Regions. In this way a method for establishing good practice can be set up and monitored which can be used to develop standards and interact with management, research and development, and education in order to improve care. The managers in the provider units use the audit process to identify deficiencies and rectify them as part of the quality assurance and control process. Identifying care outcomes is not as easy as it may seem because while some of the outcomes are very easy to assess, e.g. diagnosis of fetal abnormalities others such as backache after delivery are not so obvious. Having said this, audit is a very good way of monitoring actual clinical care and is an essential part of the measurement of its effectiveness and is one of the main ways that clinical care can be assessed by both purchasers and providers.

The rationale for monitoring and audit is to improve care and ensure that it is effective, that there is equity, access acceptability, efficiency and effective use of resources. This being so it is an agent for change and should ensure that the spirit of 'Changing Childbirth' is made a reality and women will be assured of a maternity service focused on their needs and one in which they are active participants and partners in their care, having choice, continuity and control.

CHAPTER EIGHT

Research and Education

In order to improve the service provided to women current practice must be evaluated and midwives should be encouraged to undertake research into their own practice. While not all midwives will be involved in the research process every practising midwife must be capable of evaluating her own practice in the light of current research. Midwives must also be equipped to give care which is based on knowledge of the many factors which affect women and their lives.

The importance of education and research to the overall standard of care was acknowledged within the 'Changing Childbirth' Report (Department of Health, 1993a) with the stipulation of two objectives which should be met:

1. Staff should receive training to enable them to support all women with different needs to that they can use the service to maximum advantage. (p.58)
2. Clinical practice should be based on sound evidence and be subject to regular clinical audit. (p. 64)

If midwives are to contribute effectively and equally to the provision of maternity care then it is important that they are prepared to undertake this role. How midwives are educated will influence their ability and enthusiasm to offer a service which is enabling and supportive as well as their capacity to review care critically with reference to new knowledge and current research. Preparation of midwives to undertake their full role needs to be addressed both within basic and continuing education programmes. But where, how and by whom education is provided will influence any attempts to educate and develop the midwives required to undertake the role demanded by 'Changing Childbirth'. It may be relevant, therefore to reflect on the present state of midwifery education.

Midwifery education

Within the United Kingdom, midwifery education has moved away from its clinical base and amalgamated with schools of nursing into higher education establishments. While the benefits have been extolled, for example, interprofessional learning and research opportunities (Henderson, 1994), there is no evidence that research activity is actually increased to date (Crotty, 1993) and presently the main thrust of interprofessional learning is between nurses and midwives. The opportunity of sharing learning with other groups is necessarily curtailed by the absence of other health care professionals within many higher education establishments.

The greatest danger of the changes is the dissolution of the ties between educationalists and practitioners which are affected not only by the physical movement of teachers into distant colleges of higher education and the emphasis on academic activity of the teachers (Dickinson, 1994) but also by the requirements of the new courses. In the main, most teaching sessions have to be newly planned and prepared. For a one hour teaching session, a period of two to three hours preparation is not uncommon. All these factors have resulted in midwife teachers spending less time within the clinical areas.

While it is acknowledged that some teachers may welcome the opportunity to further their academic profile, it is not necessarily a desirable outcome for the profession. Warwick (1992) states that:

> 'midwifery is, and will always be, fundamentally a practice based profession. It is only by valuing and giving credit to this practice that we will both establish our right to our own identity in the wider education arena and retain that which has always been midwifery's greatest strength – the total integration of education and practice'.

The challenge for educators is to ensure that all courses are midwifery led and that practice is integrated and applied to all aspects of the curriculum.

Having a programme that is midwifery led may be open to many interpretations, from courses that are designed and delivered by midwife teachers to others which are managerially controlled by a midwife but delivered by lecturers from different departments of the college or university, or delivered within other departments of the college. This fragmentation of curriculum delivery is more likely where education programmes are divided into modules.

In higher education a modular approach to delivery of courses is common practice. Each education programme is divided into a series of subjects or themes taught over a one semester or two semester period, with on average three to four hours teacher contact per module per week. Modules may cover a range of themes from ethics to biological studies. With the practice of shared learning, student midwives are usually in the minority, the danger is that any subjects may have a nursing focus, or as Kent et al (1994) found, lack midwifery application. This may be inevitable because, in the search for greater and greater depth, the subject will, of necessity, be delivered by a specialist. The fact that midwifery is a cohesive discipline drawn from many subjects may be lost in this quest for subject specialization.

This approach has its champions, Page (1993) suggests that subjects which underpin midwifery practice should be delivered by specialist lecturers with midwives, either teachers or practitioners, teaching midwifery and the relevance of specialist subjects to practice. For those with practical midwifery experience this may appear an obvious solution, but for the student with limited practical knowledge the danger may be that the theory practice gap may be replaced by a theory-theory gap. What appears to be forgotten is that in order for a teacher to apply the theory to professional practice, he or she must have sufficient knowledge of the original subject. In many instances this knowledge may be sufficient to allow the teacher to integrate both the specialist knowledge and implications for practice and thereby prevent unnecessary duplication of teaching.

In their review of pre-registration midwifery Stark and Elzubeir (1994) state that there was a shortcoming on the part of the students in understanding the relevance of, assimilating and applying specialist input to midwifery. They do not appear to have explored totally why this occurred, but it may be that those with no experience of midwifery lack the ability to apply theories to make them relevant to midwifery and are consequently not of interest to the student. It may also be that midwife teachers are under such pressure to generalize that they are not developing their own skills in synthesizing the knowledge that is delivered.

Jackson (1994) equates the use of specialist lectures and supplementary sessions with the past practice of compulsory consultant lectures which required midwife teacher application and interpretation. If this practice was rejected on the grounds that midwives should have control over their own education why has it now been deemed acceptable that a considerable proportion of midwifery education can be provided by other specialists? Perhaps the midwifery profession as a whole should heed the warning of Margaret Brain issued in 1989 'as a profession we have the right to control and assess or own education and it is essential that we do so. In fact if we lose control of our education we lose control of our profession' (cited by Warwick, 1992). The recommendation of Winterton (House of Commons, 1992) that midwifery education be delivered in faculties of midwifery seems to have been forgotten.

The preparation of midwives to meet the recommendations of 'Changing Childbirth' (Department of Health, 1993a) requires an application of the physical, social, psychological and cultural factors which influence the health, wellbeing and status of women. Is it not feasible that the best people to help midwives develop their knowledge and assist them in applying such knowledge to midwifery are those within their own profession?

Applying theory to actual practice situations, however, cannot be achieved within the classroom. Whereas practising midwives have the clinical experience to assist them apply new knowledge to their practice, student midwives need the help of experienced and knowledgeable practitioners who have the time and commitment to undertake this role. Practitioners can argue that workload sometimes inhibit the process and it must be acknowledged that some midwives may lack the willingness or relevant knowledge to undertake this important role. Midwife teachers have traditionally seen clinical teaching as part of their role, although, as previously stated, there is some evidence that this has reduced with the changes in education (Dickinson, 1994). Teacher involvement in practice is acknowledged by midwives as an important factor in assisting integration of theory and practice (Henderson, 1994; Page, 1993) and by students who see teachers as the people who know their present depth of knowledge and can help them apply that knowledge within the clinical areas (Raymond and Ananda-Rajan, 1993). If this is not enough encouragement for teachers to become involved clinically, they should consider the Midwife's Code of Practice (UKCC, 1994a) and the Department of Health publication, 'A Strategy for Nursing' (1989). The Midwife's Code of Practice (UKCC, 1994a) states that practising midwives must take responsibility for maintaining and developing their practice and acquiring competence in new skills. This should not be interpreted by the midwife teacher solely as educational skills. If clinicians are required to keep up to date in theory is it not fair that teachers should also be required to update on clinical advancements? A Strategy for Nursing (Department of Health, 1989) state that teachers must be able to demonstrate at an advanced level a knowledge of theory *and* practice.

Page (1993) suggests the extension of the role of lecturer practitioner as a way of integrating education and practice, but experiments with this role within nursing has led to some dilemmas for the lecturer practitioner. Burke (1993) argues that conflict between the needs of the learner and the needs of the patient can occur, being answerable to two masters both of whom can have very different expectations of the role can cause some degree of stress for the lecturer practitioner. There is no reason to expect that similar problems do not or would not occur within midwifery. This is not to say that the idea should be abandoned, but clear guidelines to the expectations of the role would have to be agreed, and as Burke (1993) points out the introduction of self-governing trusts together with the movement of education into higher education institutions would make such agreements difficult.

The model introduced by the midwife teachers in North London College of Health Studies (Dickinson, 1994) appears a more workable approach. Midwife teachers are committed to 45 days per year clinical involvement. This is divided into 25 days for student contact, 10 days for clinical support activities and 10 days for individual clinical practice. The latter is usually undertaken in one two-week block or two one-week blocks. Some problems have been identified, mainly with balancing other educational demands. It does appear that this system is one way of ensuring that students are supported and taught within the clinical areas, and the teachers themselves are retaining practical midwifery knowledge. Another way may be to devise a new model whereby the teacher functions as a member of the care team, if only for planned periods of time.

In whatever way the problem of integrating theory and practice is resolved it is important that the profession as a whole addresses the issues and solutions are found which will ensure that the training and education of midwives remains under professional control and retains its clinical focus.

Basic education programmes

There are currently three main types of programmes of education and training for admission to Part 10 of the UKCC Register; a three-year course with academic credit at Diploma of Higher Education level; a four-year degree programme; and a 78-week programme for registered nurses also at diploma of higher education academic level. It is not intended to discuss the merits or otherwise of these various programmes but to consider how curricula may need to be revised to provide the midwife of the future.

If this is to occur programme planners will need to take into account the changes in practice. Students will be allocated to a team of midwives for the entire period of training and while the advantages are enormous in that the student will see the total role of the midwife, there are implications for the theoretical input. Most programmes start from a basis of normality progressing to the pathological conditions which complicate pregnancy, with the clinical allocation mirroring the theoretical input. In the future midwifery programmes will have to reflect the more holistic approach to care.

The curriculum model suggested by Donovan and Duckett (1994) acknowledges that abnormal conditions can be encountered at any time during clinical experience and attempts to incorporate information regarding such conditions throughout the programme, but they have not addressed the allocation of students to a team of midwives. Their curriculum retains the traditional model of clinical allocation to a specific area with theoretical content reflecting the clinical experience.

Regardless of theway the curriculum is arranged there is the need to address the skills required by the midwife in the future. Page (1993) identifies a 'triangle of skills', these are intellectual, personal and clinical. How these skills are combined to develop midwives, 'capable of using clinical judgment, of making clinical decisions, of carrying and organising a caseload, of high interpersonal communication skills and ... [have] considerable manual dexterity' (Page, 1993) is an important issue for any midwifery programme and integrating them throughout the course is essential. Along with developing an understanding of the physiological processes of childbearing, the curriculum must address the social, cultural and political context of childbearing and midwifery care, and the interpersonal skills required for effective relationship building and multiprofessional team cooperation. Including these skills with a modular programme may be the answer, but they must be identified as core compulsory modules and skills developed must be integrated throughout the programme.

Developing the skills of critical thinking and evaluation of practice is an essential component of any education programme in order that midwives are equipped to take responsibility for their future development needs. This can be achieved in two ways, which are equipping students with the ability to evaluate practice in the light of current research and promoting independent learning. Many of the current education programmes include these skills, but unless they are evident within practice there is a danger that newly qualified midwives will become disenchanted with practice or lose enthusiasm to develop their skills throughout their working lives.

For midwives currently in practice the opportunity to develop new skills, both practical and intellectual can be provided by planned continuing education programmes but these must be both relevant and accessible.

Continuing education

The Expert Group (Department of Health, 1993a) acknowledge the importance of education and training by stating 'staff education and training is a key element in meeting the diversity of women's needs', and stipulating that, 'Providers, statutory and professional bodies should ensure that all staff have access to training which is designed to help them understand the differing needs women may have' (pp. 57 and 58). The Report also identifies some of the skills which need to be developed, i.e. resuscitation and examination and care of the newborn. It is important that both local and national consideration is given to the requirements of midwives both for the short and long-term. The Department of Health and Royal College of Midwives have made available funds for the appointment of a midwife to assess the implications for training of 'Changing Childbirth', but there is much that can be done locally to assist midwives adapt to their new role.

The Report states that 'for the majority of women pregnancy and birth will be uncomplicated' (p. 12) and this may be a useful starting point for midwives whose experience of hospital based care and intervention may have distorted their image of pregnancy and labour to one of high-risk which is only normal in retrospect. Midwives may need to revisit the physiological process involved and identify how they can support this process. Study days and weeks which are attended as part of periodic refreshment requirements could be used to explore these and other issues. The importance of addressing basic knowledge should not be underestimated. For example, to review the physiology of labour with the experience of many years of caring for women can be a tremendously enlightening experience as many who have undertaken further academic study will testify. It can also help to progress to explore the wider issues, for example the effect of psychological and cultural factors on the physiological processes. Giving midwives confidence in their skills is essential and it is only by revisiting some of the basics and building upon them that this confidence can be fostered.

The need to expand interpersonal skills is emphasized throughout the report. On the personal level there is the need to improve communication between the midwife and the women. Midwives need to develop ways to encourage women to convey their wishes regarding care. Many women, not used to being consulted, need encouragement, empathy and information to make decisions. Giving unbiased information is another skill which midwives need to perfect.

On an organizational level midwives need to prepare to work within a team. Along with team building and leadership skills, the role of the lead professional must be addressed. Midwives need to explore the expectations of the role and how it fits with the multiprofessional approach to care. For the future, organizational skills may be important. Purchasing and contracting may need to be included along with setting up a group practice.

The issue of developing new practical skills has been addressed to some degree. Skills already developed in some units include: siting of intravenous cannulae, giving intravenous drugs, prescribing postoperative analgesia and ultrasound scanning (Spence-Jones, 1994). The reasons given for increasing the repertoire of midwifery skills is the enhancement of holistic care and the result of the reduction in junior doctor hours. One can speculate on the future and ask whether or not other practices will be included, for instance forceps delivery? The inclusion of such a task may be seen as desirable by some within the profession either in the name of holistic care or development of advanced midwifery practice or clinical specialist role.

The United Kingdom Central Council in its recent paper setting out standards for education and practice following registration defines advanced midwifery practice 'pioneering and developing of new roles responsive to changing needs and with advancing clinical practice, research and education' (UKCC, 1994b, p. 22). They also acknowledge that studies for advanced midwifery practice are likely to be at Masters level. Whether or not the new roles of advancing clinical practice will include such skills as forceps delivery has not been addressed. If, in the future they are included, not all midwives will develop such skills, and the vision of a midwife who has not previously been involved in the care of a woman being called to undertake a forceps delivery leads back to the question: what is midwifery? The Association of Radical Midwives in its response to 'Changing Childbirth' (Warren, 1993) has identified the need to develop skill and competency in the management of home births. Many midwives have little or no experience in caring for women at home and in dealing with emergencies in the home environment. They recommend the development of a programme where those with the expertise, for example independent midwives and those within established teams, can disseminate their knowledge and offer practical training and advice to colleagues.

One issue concerning the education of midwives to meet the requirements of the future, is that of assessment of their competence. The Midwife's Code of Practice (UKCC, 1994a) requires that each midwife is responsible to develop new skills and the Supervisor of midwives role in ensuring that midwives gain the experience and education necessary to fulfil new aspects of her role is explicit.

How will competency be assessed and if midwives fail to reach the competency required can they be deemed incapable of fulfilling the role of the midwife? The Midwife's Code of Practice (UKCC, 1994b) gives some guidance regarding the development of new skills which do not necessarily become an integral part of the role of the midwife by stating 'each employing authority should have locally agreed policies which observe the Council's requirements and National Board advice and guidelines.' (p. 10). There is no guidance for the development of skills and expertise of managing home delivery which may be lost or never gained because of lack of opportunity during initial training.

The Report acknowledges that the role of the Senior House Officer (SHO) needs to be reviewed with emphasis on the training aspects rather than service commitments, and that this will have implications for midwives and senior obstetricians (p. 42). For midwives it is not only their clinical role that will be required to change, they may be required to undertake a more active role in the education of junior obstetric staff and general practitioner trainees. There is no clear indication as to the status of the midwives who will be required to undertake teaching of the SHO.

It is not only the actual training of these doctors that need to be addressed, but how and by whom their competence will be assessed. Currently there is no formal method of assessment of these practitioners, but if a structured approach to their training is implemented it is feasible that their ability to meet the clinical requirements could be introduced. If the emphasis is on normal childbrith then the most obvious person to assess competency is the person most experienced in the assessment of normality, i.e. the midwife. This issue will need to be addressed by both the medical and midwifery professions.

Research

The introduction of practices which are not backed-up by research evidence is highlighted by 'Changing Childbirth' (DOH, 1993a), echoing the sentiments of Enkin et al (1989). There is a need not only that research is undertaken by midwives, but that research data and reports are readily available to them and they have the skills to appraise the reports.

The importance of midwives being involved in research is examined by Allison and Tyler (1994) who acknowledge that midwives, although fairly new to the research arena, have proved to have a profound effect on practice, not only in altering procedures but in examining the effect of interactions between women and midwives. It is now vitally important that midwives become more involved in evaluating any changes implemented to attain the targets recommended by 'Changing Childbirth' (DOH, 1993a). Many of the recommendations have a 'feel right' factor, but this is not a secure enough base on which to change practice. Evaluation needs to be undertaken on a local basis as well as nationally, and midwives need the support to conduct such studies. Time to pursue such activities is essential and financial help is needed.

There are many funds available to midwives to assist with their research activities. The Royal College of Midwives offers yearly scholarships to midwives wishing to undertake research projects and many of our current well known researchers have used this fund as a springboard into research. The English National Board for Nursing, Midwifery and Health Visiting fund many research projects and have recently invited the professionals to 'identify areas, issues and questions which they consider to be important and deserving of priority for research' (ENB, 1994). Regional Health Authorities also contribute financially to research initiatives and the Department of Health has recently appointed a midwife to evaluate the projects funded to improve maternity care within the recommendations of 'Changing Childbirth'.

It is also important that midwives are involved in multidisciplinary research projects. The National Perinatal and Epidemiology Unit has demonstrated the way forward in this field, but there is the need for more such units in other parts of the country. The establishment of midwifery education within institutes of higher education may assist the development of collaborative studies with other disciplines such as the social scientists many of whom have contributed much to the understanding of the social implications of childbearing.

The action points detailed by 'Changing Childbirth' are themselves areas where research could be initiated. These include:

1. Accessible services – how can this be achieved to the satisfaction of the women.
2. Information giving – what methods are most appropriate to women.
3. The named midwife – a comparison between the midwives' and women's perceptions.
4. Lead professional – implications for women and professionals.
5. Making choices – the effect of social, cultural and professional factors on women making choices.
6. Flexible systems of care – effectiveness and efficiency of such systems.
7. Place of birth – implications of accommodating individual choice.

'Changing Childbirth' concluded that:

> 'there is much that is good in maternity care in this country, but it is also clear that further reform is both desirable and inevitable. The changes set out in this report represent a move towards more woman-centred care in which users will be able to take part in decision making about their own care and provide feedback about their experiences to improve the services of the future' (p. 106).

It is important that these views are sought, but also that the professionals continue to assess practice so that all care offered can be demonstrated to be for the benefit of the women and their babies and that they become the focus of care which is proven to be of benefit and in keeping with their wishes.

References

Alexander, S., Keirse, M.J.N.C. (1989). 'Formal risk scoring during pregnancy'. In: Enkin, M.W., Keirse, M.J.N.C., Chalmers, I. (Eds). *Effective Care in Pregnancy and Childbirth*. Oxford: Oxford University Press, pp 345–65.

Allison, J., Tyler, S. (1994). 'How to ensure research-based practice.' In: Chamberlain, G., Patel, N. (Eds.) *The Future of the Maternity Services*. London: RCOG Press. pp. 276–81.

Association of Radical Midwives (1986). *The Vision. Proposals for the Future of the Maternity Services*. Ormskirk: ARM.

Ball, J.A., Flint, C., Garvey, M., Jackson-Baker, A., Page, L. (1992). *Who's Left Holding the Baby?* Leeds: The Nuffield Institute for Health Services Studies.

Bower, H. (1993). 'Team Midwifery in Oxford'. *MIDIRS Midwifery Digest* 3, 2, pp.143-45.

Brooks, L., Black, M. (1994). 'Local delivery (the women of the London borough of Redbridge answer a questionnaire on what they want from the maternity services)'. *Health Service Journal*, Feb. 10, p.33.

Burke, L.M. (1993). 'The future of the Specialist Nurse Teacher: Two different models explained'. *Nurse Education Today* 13, pp. 40–46.

Campbell, R., MacFarlane, A.J. (1987). *Where to be Born? The Debate and the Evidence*. Oxford: National Perinatal Epidemiology Unit.

Chamberlain, G. and Patel, N. (Eds). (1994). *The Future of the Maternity Services*. London: Royal College of Obstetricians and Gynaecologists Press.

Charles, J. (1993). 'Team Midwifery'. *Midwives Chronicle*, May, p.146.

Cornwell, J. (1984). *Hard Earned Lives*. London: Tavistock Publications.

Crottty, M. (1993). 'The changing role of the nurse teacher.' *Nurse Education Today*. 13 pp. 415–20.

Demilew, J. (1994). 'South East London Midwifery Group Practice'. *MIDIRS Midwifery Digest* 4, 3, pp.270-72.

Department of Employment (1974). *Health and Safety At Work Act*. London: HMSO.

Department of Health (1982). *Patient's First*. London: HMSO.

Department of Health (1989). *A Strategy for Nursing*. London: HMSO.

Department of Health (1989). *Women's experiences of maternity care – A Survey Manual: Office of Population, Censuses and Surveys*. London: HMSO.

Department of Health (1989). *Working for Patients*. London: HMSO.

Department of Health (1990a). *NHS and Community Care Act*. London: HMSO.

Department of Health (1990b). *An Introductory Guide to the Children Act for the NHS*. London: HMSO.

Department of Health (1991). *The Patient's Charter*. London: HMSO.

Department of Health (1992a). *The Health of the Nation*. London: HMSO.

Department of Health (1992b). *Maternity Services. Government Response to the Second Report from the Health Committee Session 91–92*. London: HMSO.

Department of Health (1993a). *Changing Childbirth The Report of the Expert Maternity Group*. London: HMSO.

Department of Health (1993b). *The Health of the Nation – Key Area Handbook: Mental Illness*. London: HMSO.

Department of Health (1993c). *NHS Management Exectuive Letter* EL(93)72. London: DOH.

Department of Health (1993d). *Clinical Audit*. London: HMSO.

Department of Health (1994). *The Patient's Charter: The Maternity Services*. London: HMSO.

Department of Health (1994). *Nursing Strategy Workshop. 'Health and Social Care 2010, Shaping the Future'. The Challenges for Nursing and Midwifery in the 21st Century: The Heathrow Debate*. London: HMSO.

Dickinson, A. (1994). 'Clinical involvement of midwife teachers.' *Nursing Standard*. 8:25 pp.25–30.

Dimond, B. (1994). 'Midwifery Managed Units'. *Modern Midwife,* June, pp.31–33.

Donabedian, A. (1969). 'Quality care: Problems of Measurement, Part 2 Some Issues of Evaluating the Quality of Nursing Care'. *Journal of Public Health* Vol. 59, pp. 1833–36.

Donovan, P., Duckett, M. (1994). 'The southampton wave' *Modern Midwife*. June pp.15–16.

Dunlop, W. (1993). 'Changing Childbirth – Commentary II'. *British Medical Journal* 100, pp.1072–74.

English National Board (1994). 'Nursing, Midwifery and Health Visiting Education. A systematic approach to identify research and development (R & D) priorities'. *Education and Practice*, November.

Enkin, N.W., Keirse, M.J.N.C., Chalmers, I. (1989). *Effective Care in Pregnancy and Childbearing*. Oxford: Oxford University Press.

Fawdrey, R (1994). 'Antenatal case Notes 1: Comments on Design'. *British Journal of Midwifery,* July, Vol .2, No. 7, pp 320–27.

Fawdrey, R (1994). 'Antenatal case Notes 2: General comments'. *British Journal of Midwifery* August, Vol. 2, No. 8, pp 371–74.

Flint, C. (1993). *Midwifery Teams and Caseloads*. London: Butterworth Heinemann.

Garcia, J. (1987). 'The role and structure of the MSLC. ' *Health Trends* Vol. 19, pp. 17–19.

Garcia, J., Blondell, B., Saurel-Cubizolles, M.J. (1989). "The needs of childbearing families: social policies and organisation of health care'. In: Enkin, N.W., Keirse, M.J.N.C., Chalmers, I. (Eds). *Effective Care in Pregnancy and Childbearing*. Oxford: Oxford University Press, pp205–20.

Gill, S (1994). 'Safety at all hours'. *Modern Midwife,* July, p 28–30.

Guelbert, C. (1994). Progress report on Project Liverbirth. Unpublished. October. Liverpool Health Authorities.

Hall, H.M., Chng, P.K., MacGillivray, I. (1980). 'Is routine antenatal care worthwhile?' *Lancet* ii, pp.78–80.

Hamilton, P.M. (1994). *An Ethnographic Study of Postnatal Care in the Community*.M.Sc. Unpublished Dissertation, Keele University.

Heelas, P., Morris, P. (1992). 'The value of the enterprise culture' In: Heelas, P., Morris, P.(Eds). *The Values of the Enterprise Culture* London: Routledge.

Helman, C.G. (1990). *Culture Health and Illness*.. London: Butterworth-Heinemann.

Henderson, C. (1994). 'The education and training of midwives' In Chamberlain, G., Patel, N. (Eds) *The Future of the Maternity services*. London: RCOG Press. pp. 220–27.

HMSO (1989). *Working for Patients. Self Governing Hospitals: An initial Guide*. A paper for a national conference. 29 June 1989 London: HMSO.

House of Commons (1955–56). The Report of the Committee of Inquiry into the Cost of the National Health Service – The Obstetric Service under the National Health Service. Chairman: Guillebaud. London: HMSO.

House of Commons (1979–80). *Social Services Committee, Second Report, Perinatal and Neonatal Mortality.* Chairman: Short., R. London:HMSO.

House of Commons (1991–92). *Health Committee, Second Report, Maternity Services.* Chairman: Winterton, N. London: HMSO.

House of Commons (1992). *Maternity Services: Government Response to the Second Report from the Health Committee, Session 1991–92.* London: HMSO.

Institute of Manpower Studies (1993). *Mapping Team Midwifery.* IMS Report Series, 242.

Jackson, K. (1994). 'Knowing Your Midwife: How easy is it?' *British Journal of Midwifery,* October, Vol 2, No.10, pp.507–508.

Kent, J., MacKeith, N., Maggs, C. (1994). *Direct, but difficult; an evaluation of the implementation of pre-registration midwifes in England.* London: Crown Publications.

Kirkham, M. (1989). 'Midwives and information giving during labour'. In: Robinson, S., Thomson, A.M. (Eds). *Midwives, Research and Childbirth* Vol. 1. London: Chapman Hall.

Kitzinger, S. (1989). 'Childbirth and society'. In: Enkin, M., Keirse, M.J.N.C., Chalmers, I. (Eds). *Effective Care in Pregnancy and Childbirth..* Oxford: Oxford University Press, pp99–109.

Kitzinger, S. (1991). *Homebirth and Other Alternatives to Hospital.* London: Dorling Kindersley.

Klein, M., Lloyd, I., Redman, C., Bull, M., Turnbull, A.C. (1983). 'A comparison of low risk pregnant women booked for delivery in two systems of care'. *Br. J. Obstet & Gynaecol.* 90, pp.118–22.

Lee, G. (1994). 'A reassuring family face?'. *Nursing Times* April 27, 90, 17, pp. 66–67.

Lewison, H. (1994). *Maternity Services Liaison Committees: A Forum for Change.* Greater London: Association of Community Health Councils/National Childbirth Trust

Marsh, J., Sargent, E. (1991). 'Factors affecting the duration of postnatal visits'. *Midwifery* 7, pp.177–82.

Martin, E. (1987). *The Woman in the Body.* Milton Keynes: Open University Press.

Maternity Advisory Committee (1970). *Domiciliary and Maternity Bed Needs.* Chairman: Peel, Sir John. London: HMSO.

Maternity Services Advisory Committee (1982). *Maternity Care in Action, Part 1– Antenatal Care.* London: HMSO.

Maternity Services Advisory Committee (1984). *Materntiy Care in Action, Part 2– Care During Childbirth.* London: HMSO.

Maternity Services Advisory Committee (1985). *Maternity Care in Action Part 3 – Care of the Mother and Baby.* London: HMSO.

McCrea, H., Crute, V. (1994). 'Midwife/client relationships: midwives' perspectives'. *Midwifery* 7, pp.183–92.

Mclean, G. (1994). 'Safe motherhood in the United Kingdom'. *Modern Midwife* June, pp.10–14.

Methven, R. (1989). 'Recording an obstetric history or relating to a pregnant woman? A Study of the anteantal booking interview'. In: Robinson, S. and Thompson, A. (Eds). *Midwives, Research and Childbirth* 1(4), pp 42–71. London: Chapman Hall.

Morris-Thompson, P. (1994). 'Contracting for Maternity Services'. *MIDIRS Midwifery Digest* Vol 4, No 2, June, pp 232–33.

Murphy-Black, T. (1992). 'Systems of midwifery care in use in Scotland' *Midwifery* 8, pp.112–24.

Murphy-Black, T. (1993). 'Home birth: can we offer women choices for childbirth?' *British Journal of Midwifery* 1, 4, pp 166–69.

Namelle, N., Laumon, B. (1984). 'Occupational fatigue and preterm birth'. In: Chamberlain, G. (Ed). *Pregnant Women at Work.* London: Macmillan.

NHS (1989). *Review Working Paper 1: Self Governing Hospitals.* London: HMSO.

NHS Management Executive (1993). *Risk Management in the NHS.* London: DOH.

Oakley, A. (1992). 'Social support in pregnancy: Methodology and findings of a one year follow-up study'. *J. Reproductive and Inf. Psychol.* 10:4 pp.219–31.

Oakley, A. (1993). *Essays on Women, Medicine and Health.* Edinburgh: Edinburgh University Press.

Oakley, A., Houd, S. (1990). *Helpers in Childbirth Midwifery Today* London: Hemisphere Publishing Corporation.

Page, L (1994). 'Professional alliances: some of my best friends' *Midwives Chronicle,* Jan, pp10-12.

Page, L. (1993). 'Changing childbirth: A renewal of the Maternity Services'. *British Journal of Midwifery* September, Vol 1, No. 4, p.157.

Page, L. (1993). 'Education for practice' *MIDIRS Midwifery Digest* 3:3 pp. 253–56.

Page, L., Jones, B., Bentley, R,. Cooke, P,. Harding, M., Stevens, T,. Wilkins, R. (1994). 'One-to-one Midwifery Practice'. *British Journal of Midwifery* 2, 9, pp.444-47.

Patterson, L., Burns, J. (1990). *Women, Assertiveness and Health.* London: Health Education Authority.

Pill, R., Stott, N. (1991). 'Concepts of illness causation and responsibility: some preliminary data from a sample of working class mothers'. In: Currer, C., Stacey, M. (Eds). *Concepts of Health, Illness and Disease.* Oxford: Sage.

Popay, J. (1992). 'My health is all right, but I'm just tired all the time: women's experiences of ill health'. In: Roberts, H. (Ed) *Women's Health Matters.* London: Routledge.

Raymond, J., Ananda-Rajan, K. (1993). 'Learning practice' *Nursing Times.* 89:31 pp.36-37.

Royal College of Midwives (1987). *Towards a Healthy Nation A Policy for the Maternity Services.* London: RCM.

Royal College of Midwives (1993). *Good Practice Guidelines for MSLCs.* London: RCM.

Royal College of Obstetricians and Gynaecologists (1982). *Report of the RCOG Working Party on Antenatal and Intrapartum Care* September, London: RCOG.

Royal College of Obstetricians and Gynaecologists (1992). *Maternity Care in the New NHS. A Joint Approach.* London: RCOG.

Royal College of Obstetricians and Gynaecologists (1993). *Changing Childbirth Report of the Expert Group on Maternity Services.* Press release August 6th.

Sandelowski, M. (1994). 'Separate, but less equal; fetal ultrasonography and the transformation of the expectant mother/ fatherhood'. *Gender and Society* 8:2, pp. 230–45.

Schott, J. (1994). 'The importance of encouraging women to think for themselves'. *British Journal of Midwifery* 2, 1, pp. 3–4.

SpenceJones, C. (1994). 'Labour forces.' *Nursing Times.* 90:3 pp. 70–71.

Stacey, M. (1976). 'The health service consumer: a sociological misconception'. *Soc. Rev. Monographs.* 22, pp.194–200.

Stark, S., Elzuber, M. (1994) 'Effects of the lack of nurse training on pre-registration midwifery students.' *British Journal of Midwifery.* 2:4 pp.182–86.

Stirrat, G.M. (1988). 'Risk arising during pregnancy.' In: James, D.K., Stirrat, G.M. (Eds). *_Pregnancy and Risk the Basis for Rational Management.* Chichester: John Wiley & Sons.

Stock J. (1993). 'Providing Continuity –the Experience of Midwives'. *Midwives Chronicle,* Dec. p.476.

Strathern, M. (1992). 'Enterprise kinship: Consumer choice in the new reproductive technologies'. In: Heelas, P., Morris, P. (Eds). *The Values of the Enterprise Culture.* London: Routledge.

Tew, M. (1990). *Safer Childbirth? A Critical History of Maternity Care.* London: Chapman and Hall.

The Challenges of Nursing and Midwifery in the 21st Century (1993). *The Heathrow Debate.* London: HMSO.

Tyler, S and Jenkins, R. (1994). 'Can GPs reach the high Cs?' *Health Service Journal*, January, p.30.

UCL Hospitals, Women's Health Directorate Maternity Services (1994). Equal Access Policy and Code of Practice. Unpublished.

UKCC (16/1994). *Position Statement on Waterbirth.* Registrar's Letter. 6 October.

United Kingdom Central Council for Nursing, Midwifery and Health Visiting (1993). *Midwives Rules.* November. London: UKCC.

United Kingdom Central Council for Nursing, Midwifery and Health Visiting (1994). *The Midwife's Code of Practice.* May. London: UKCC.

United Kingdom Central Council for Nursing, Midwifery and Health Visiting (1994a). *The Future of Professional Practice -the Council's Standards for Education and Practice following Registration.* London: UKCC.

United Kingdom Central Council for Nursing, Midwifery and Health Visiting (1994b). *The Midwife's Code of Practice.* London: UKCC.

United Kingdom Central Council for Nursing, Midwifery and Health Visiting. (1992). *Code of Professional Conduct for Nurses, Midwives and Health Visitors.* London: UKCC.

United Kingdom Central Council for Nursing, Midwifery and Health Visiting. (1992). *Community Postnatal Visiting. Registrar's Letter No. 11.* London: UKCC.

Ward, P., Frohlich, J. (1994). Team Midwifery in Bristol. *MIDIRS Midwifery Digest* 4, 2, pp.149-51.

Wardle, S (1994). 'Getting Consumers' Views of Maternity Services'. *Professional Care of Mother and Child* August, pp.170–74.

Warren, C., Hughes, D., Bowman, L., Kargar, I. (1993). 'ARMs response to changing childbirth.' *Midwifery Matters*, 59, p.4.

Warwick, C. (1992). 'Reflections on the current management of midwifery education'. *MIDIRS*, 23, p. 251–54.

Indicators of Success

Within five years

1. All women should be entitled to carry their own notes.

2. Every woman should know one midwife who ensures continuity of her midwifery care – the named midwife.

3. At last 30 per cent of women should have the midwife as the lead professional.

4. Every woman should know the lead professional who has a key role in the planning and provision of her care.

5. At least 75 per cent of women should know the person who cares for them during their delivery.

6. Midwives should have direct access to some beds in all maternity units.

7. At least 30 per cent of women delivered in a maternity unit should be admitted under the management of the midwife.

8. The total number of antenatal visits for women with uncomplicated pregnancies should have been reviewed in the light of the available evidence and the RCOG guidelines.

9. All front line ambulances should have a paramedic able to support the midwife who needs to transfer a woman to hospital in an emergency.

10. All women should have access to information about the services available in their locality.

Index